Contributions to Psychology a

Christine Eiser

The Psychology
of Childhood Illness

Springer-Verlag
New York Berlin Heidelberg Tokyo

Christine Eiser
Department of Psychology
University of Exeter
Exeter EX4 4QG
England

Advisor
J. Richard Eiser
Department of Psychology
University of Exeter
Exeter EX4 4QG
England

Library of Congress Cataloging in Publication Data
Eiser, Christine.
  The psychology of childhood illness.
  (Contributions to psychology and medicine)
  Bibliography: p.
  Includes index.
  1. Pediatrics—Psychological aspects.
  2. Sick children—Psychology. I. Title. II. Series
  RJ47.5.E37   1985   618.92'0001'9   84-23577

Typeset by Ampersand Publisher Services, Inc., Rutland, Vermont.
Printed and bound by R.R. Donnelley & Sons Company,
Harrisonburg, Virginia.
Printed in the United States of America.

9 8 7 6 5 4 3 2 1

ISBN 0-387-96096-1 Springer-Verlag New York Berlin Heidelberg Tokyo
ISBN 3-540-96096-1 Springer-Verlag Berlin Heidelberg New York Tokyo

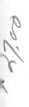

for David and Benjamin

Preface

The pattern of childhood illness has changed significantly during this century. Many frightening conditions such as polio and tuberculosis have essentially been eradicated. Other conditions that were once fatal have now achieved the status of chronic disorders, for example, leukemia, cancer, and cystic fibrosis. Technological advances which have resulted in the medical treatment of these conditions have, however, created a gamut of psychological problems for the children and their families. Recognition of these problems has lagged behind other advances in pediatric medicine. The emergence of a specialist area of pediatric psychology (Wright, 1975) has largely been responsible for the mushrooming of research in the area.

In much early work, the emphasis was on the impact of chronic illness on children and their families. Reactions at times of greatest trauma, especially diagnosis or death, were particularly well documented. Issues relating to day-to-day aspects of child care, involving questions of discipline or protectiveness, have received much less attention. As far as the sick child is concerned, there has been much investigation of academic and intellectual development, as well as of personality changes that might accompany illness.

Shifts in emphasis in both pediatrics and psychology are resulting in changes in how the psychology of chronic childhood illness is now studied. There is increasing recognition that one of the aims of pediatric medicine is to ensure the cooperation of the patient and the family with the pediatrician. Any long-term management of disease is unlikely to be successful unless such cooperation is achieved. The development of such a working relationship is now seen to be dependent on the child's interpretation of the illness, its cause, and its treatment.

The contribution of developmental psychology has been to show that how a child thinks about health and illness parallels cognitive growth in other areas. Thus, the child's beliefs about the anatomy and physiology of the body, and causes and prevention of illness, are seen as developing in an orderly and systematic manner. One of the aims of this book is to show how this research, which began as a theoretical investigation of cognitive development, has profound implications for the practical care of the sick child.

The book therefore begins with an exposé of current views regarding the development of children's concepts of health and illness. Since cognitive development cannot be separated from experience, understanding of health and illness is also considered with special reference to chronically sick children. The emphasis in Chapter 2 is in showing that the way in which children interpret the cause of illness and its repercussions is largely age dependent.

Chapters 3 and 4 are concerned with general effect of illness on children. Since hospitalization is very much a part of the illness experience, considerable attention is paid to the known effects of hospital admission on children, and the effectiveness of prior pre-paration. Children's understanding of the rationale behind medical treatment is considered separately from the hospital experience. Four diseases of childhood—phenylketonuria, diabetes, leukemia, and asthma—are then considered in greater detail.

I remain indebted to the staff in the Departments of Haematology and Psychological Medicine at the Hospital for Sick Children, Great Ormond Street, London, who first gave me the opportunity to work with sick children. I am especially grateful to Mrs. Mary Lobascher who was an enthusiastic and willing teacher. Professor Philip Graham also has given much highly valued advice and encouragement. More recently, it has been a pleasure to work with Dr. J. H. Tripp and all the staff in the Pediatrics Department, Royal Devon and Exeter Hospital, Exeter. At various stages, the research on which this book is based has been funded by the Medical Research Council, the Economic and Social Research Council, and the Health Education Council of London. I am particularly indebted to Dick Eiser who has been consistently encour-aging and helpful.

Christine Eiser

Contents

Part I

Children in Health and Illness

1

Approaches to the Study of Sick Children

Advances in medical care have led to a dramatic change in the pattern of childhood disease. Improvements in sanitation and housing and the wide use of vaccinations have essentially irradicated some of the crippling disorders of the past. Diseases that are just names to a whole generation include, for example, polio and tuberculosis. Paradoxically, control of diseases such as these has not resulted in a significant decline in the absolute numbers of sick children. Advances in medicine have resulted in extended survival times for children suffering from cancer, kidney disease, and cystic fibrosis. Thus, diseases that were once fatal must now be considered chronic disorders of childhood. In addition, some children severely affected by accidents or burns can now be treated. While their injuries may have proved fatal in the past, it may often be possible to save them today. In many cases, however, treatment is likely to be lengthy and extremely painful. Such treatment may create long-term psychological problems for the child and family. As such, the challenge of caring for all these children is no longer purely medical. The purpose of this book is to consider how such long-term illness influences children's intellectual, social, and personal development.

Estimates of the incidence of chronic disorders vary. At the extreme, Stewart (1967) estimated that more than 30%–40% of children under 18 years of age suffered from one or more disorder. This figure was reached by including visual and hearing impairments, mental retardation, speech, learning and behavior disorders, as well as chronic physical conditions. Where chronic physical conditions only are included, estimates suggest that 7%–10% of children are affected (Jennison, 1976; Pless, Satterwhite, & Van Vechten, 1976; Rutter,

Tizard, & Whitmore, 1970). Mattson (1972) reported that the most common disorders were asthma (2%), epilepsy (1%), cardiac conditions (0.5%), cerebral palsy (0.5%), orthopedic illnesses (0.5%), and diabetes mellitus (0.1%). While much research attention has been given to the question of how adverse life conditions such as poor nutrition (Hoorweg & Stanfeld, 1976), inadequate caregiving (Sameroff & Chandler, 1975), or general deprivation (Madge, 1972) affect children, very much less attention has focused on the needs of chronically sick children and their families. The range of diseases and areas of research that have been investigated (Wright, 1975) are tabulated in Table 1-1.

Common sense might suggest that the diagnosis of chronic childhood disorder would inevitably have negative consequences for both the child and family. Early work very much supported this view (Robins, Bates, & O'Neil, 1962). A review of the literature by Pless and Pinkerton (1975) found evidence of problems in the child's intellectual and social functioning and potential marital and occupational status. In addition, the prognosis for normal mother–child (Shere, 1957; Turk, 1964) or marital relationships (Maguire, 1983) appeared depressing.

In attempting to describe the processes whereby chronic illness leads to such negative consequences, Stubblefield (1974) suggested that for normal children many of the natural frustrations and disappointments of growing up are overcome because there is a very realistic expectation that mastery will occur naturally with growth and development. For the chronically ill, the future is less certain. The child's sense of mastery is inhibited and this results in doubts about attaining independence and achievement. In these circumstances, chronic illness undermines normal development.

In a similar way, Hughes (1976) described eight basic emotions challenged by chronic illness: (1) love and affection, (2) security, (3) acceptance as an individual, (4) self-respect, (5) achievement, (6) recognition, (7) independence, (8) authority and discipline. Thus, for the chronically sick child, development may be influenced by rejection and lack of acceptance, hostility, and lack of affection. Day-to-day experiences may be restricted to a greater extent (as in the case of physically handicapping conditions such as cerebral palsy or thalidomide damage) or lesser extent (as with well-controlled diabetes or for children in remission from leukemia).

Yet it would be wrong to give the impression that the prognosis for the chronically sick child was so inevitably negative. Pless and Satterwhite (1975) reviewed several cases of individuals with chronic handicap, and concluded that, in some instances, greater achievements were made than might have occurred in more normal circumstances. Burton (1975) has described some children with cystic fibrosis who set out to excel in some academic pursuits while acknowledging their inability to compete with others in more physical spheres. The

Table 1-1. Childhood Diseases and Research Questions That Have Been Investigated

	Etiology	Emotional and Personality Correlates	Parental Response	Emotional and Intellectual Consequences for Child	Preparation for Medical Treatment	Health Education	Behavior Change
Congenital heart defect	—	✓	✓	✓	—	—	—
Dentistry	✓	—	—	—	✓	✓	✓
Dermatology	—	✓	—	—	—	—	✓
Endocrinology	✓	✓	✓	—	—	—	—
Gastroenterology anorexia, encopresis, lead poisoning		✓	—	—	—	—	✓
Hematology hemophilia, dying child	✓	✓	✓	✓	✓	—	—
Infectious diseases	—	✓	—	—	—	—	—
Metabolism obesity	—	—	—	—	—	✓	✓
Neonatology prematurity, crib death	✓	✓	✓	✓	—	—	—
Neurology seizures, cerebral palsy	✓	—	✓	—	—	—	✓
Orthopedics arthritis	—	—	✓	✓	—	—	—

Table 1-1. (*cont'd*)

	Etiology	Emotional and Personality Correlates	Parental Response	Emotional and Intellectual Consequences for Child	Preparation for Medical Treatment	Health Education	Behavior Change
Otorhinolaryngology cleft lip, stuttering	—	✓	—	—	—	—	✓
Psychiatry	✓	✓	—	—	—	—	✓
battered child, abused child	✓	✓	✓	—	—		
Respiratory disease (asthma cystic fibrosis)				—	—		✓
Surgery	—	—	—	✓	✓	—	—
Urology kidney transplants	—	—	✓	—	—	—	—

Adapted from Wright, L. (1975). "Pediatric psychology and problems of physical health" by L. Wright, 1975, *Journal of Clinical and Child Psychology*, Fall, 13–15.

prognosis for the family, too, may be better than originally believed. While not disputing that divorce occurs among some families with a chronically sick child, other reports suggest that families can sometimes become closer following the diagnosis (Maguire, 1983).

Clearly, the range of reactions that the child and family may make following diagnosis cover a wide spectrum. There are certain similarities between this situation and the range of outcomes identified following an aversive birth history (Lilienfeld & Parkhurst, 1951; Pasamanick & Knobloch, 1961) or inadequate caregiving (Sameroff & Chandler, 1975). These authors respectively define a "continuum of reproductive casuality" (p. 191) and a "continuum of caretaking casuality" (p. 218). In both instances, it is stressed that the prognosis for an individual subject to extremely poor or damaging circumstances is highly variable. In their original work, Lilienfeld and Parkhurst (1951) note the wide range of pregnancy outcomes, ranging from extreme conditions including cerebral palsy and epilepsy, to more subtle forms of retardation, cerebral dysfunction, and learning disability.

The repercussions for psychological development following a diagnosis of chronic childhood disorder are as varied. There is no doubt that while some children show severe mental and emotional disorders, others cope very adequately. Still others appear to function with total disregard for the illness and find it to be no apparent handicap.

There have been a number of major epidemiological studies concerned with the status of chronically sick compared with normal children. In the main, these studies point to a slightly greater risk for behavioral and emotional problems for the sick group as a whole. An early study by Keller (1953) is a case in point. Keller interviewed a random sample of families in Baltimore between 1938 and 1943. The resulting sample of 1209 children, aged between 6 and 16 years were divided into two groups; those making "satisfactory" and those making "unsatisfactory" progress. The numbers of sick children were consistently higher among those making "unsatisfactory" progress. The rates were 26.9 per 1,000 children for asthma, 12.0 per 1,000 for hay fever, 6.0 per 1,000 for heart disease, and 32.9 per 1,000 for all chronic conditions combined. In contrast, the rates for the "satisfactory" group were 17.1 per 1,000 for asthma, 5.7 per 1,000 for hay fever, and 3.4 per 1,000 for heart disease.

Three other studies are generally cited. These include the National Survey (Douglas & Blomfield, 1958), the Rochester Survey (Roghmann & Haggerty, 1970) and the Isle of Wight Survey (Rutter, Tizard & Whitmore, 1970). In the National Survey 5300 children were followed longitudinally. In the Isle of Wight study the total population of 9–11-year-old children living in the Isle of Wight was studied, and the Rochester survey included a 1% sample ($n = 1756$) of children under 18 years of age living in Monroe County, New York. In each study,

Table 1-2. Psychological Adjustment of Chronically Sick Compared With Healthy Children

All Sick Groups	Percent of Maladjusted Children						
	Isle of Wight[a]		National[b]		Rochester[c]		
	Ill	Healthy	Ill	Healthy	Age	Ill	Healthy
Parent ratings of	13.3	6.8	25	17	6–10	23	16
maladjustment					11–15	30	13
Type of illness							
Motor			23			26	
Sensory			31			44	
Cosmetic			22			35	
Duration							
Temporary			22			29	
Permanent			24			33	
Severity							
None or mild			23			27	
Moderate or			27			31	
severe							
Controls			17			16	

[a]Data from Rutter, Tizard & Whitmore, 1970.
[b]Data from Douglas & Blomfield, 1958.
[c]Data from Roghmann & Haggerty, 1970.

parental estimates of their child's adjustment were obtained by questionnaires. The results are summarized in Table 1-2, and indicate that the rates of maladjustment were higher for the chronically sick groups. It was also apparent that maladjustment rates varied as a function of the type of disorder. Children with sensory disorders tended to show higher levels of behavior problems than children with motor or cosmetic disorders, as did children with permanent rather than temporary disabilities. Those with more severe disorders showed more behavior problems than those with mild disorders, but even those with mild disorders were at greater risk of maladjustment than healthy children.

This latter finding, that even mild disorders can increase a child's psychological vulnerability, is borne out in studies of children suffering common childhood complaints. Starte (1978) investigated 204 children in a Guildford, England, practice. Illnesses occurring before 7 months of age had an adverse effect on children's developmental scores at 24 months. Orr, Weller, Satterwhite, and Pless (1984) traced 65% of the original sample of chronically sick children who had participated in the Rochester Survey. They were interviewed and also completed the California Psychological Inventory (Gough, 1975) 8 years after the initial survey. The health status of the group as a whole improved over the 8 years. For those adolescents who remained ill, however, there were several indications of poor psychosocial functioning. They often did not have a driver's license, either because of illness or parental refusal. They were less likely to be dating and more likely to have left school. Even those still in school had less clearly formulated plans for the future. Despite these findings, Orr et al. (1984) emphasize that many of the adolescents with chronic illness appear to be psychologically well. Those who had been ill in the earlier survey and were recovered by the second survey were indistinguishable from the healthy control group.

The results of the study by Orr et al. (1984) highlighted the inconsistencies in the research literature to date. While some have argued that chronic illness is associated with psychological maladjustment and that such maladjustment increases with the severity of the disease (Pless & Roghmann, 1971), others have shown greater psychological disturbance among the less severely ill (Bruhn, Hampton, & Chandler, 1971; Barker, Wright, & Myerson, 1953). Stein and Jessop (1984) further contend that the relationship between chronic illness and psychological adjustment is affected as much by demographic variables as characteristics of the illness itself. In their review of 1975, Pless and Pinkerton noted:

> Despite this formidable array of evidence remarkably little has been achieved to diminish the frequency of maladjustment among these children or more positively, to promote healthy patterns of adjustment. One explanation is that the observations and findings so far reported have not been sufficiently integrated to allow a course of intervention to be developed. (1975, p. 13)

Two major theoretical approaches have been made. Wright (1960) takes a social–psychological approach emphasizing the importance of the child's self-concept, while others (Lipowski, 1970; Mattson, 1972) emphasize the role of cognitive processes in coping behaviors. An integrated model, based on both these approaches, was developed by Pless and Pinkerton (1975).

A Social-Psychological Approach

An individual's *self-concept* needs to be distinguished from the individual's *self-esteem*. While the self-concept may be considered to be any aspect of a sense of self, including an idea of personal likes and dislikes, successes and failures, or interactions with others, self-esteem is the positive or negative value associated with the self-concept.

Wright (1960) argued that elements of self-concept differ in importance along two dimensions. The *self-connection* gradient is a description of how central each characteristic is to the individual's self-concept; the most "central"characteristics being those that define what is "really me." Some characteristics, (for example, those related to sex-role or with one's work) tend to be central for most people; others can be more individual. Wright predicted that where a physical disorder has repercussions for one of these central characteristics, there will be greater change in self-concept than if the illness affects only less central characteristics. Thus, an illness that limits a child's physical activity will have a relatively minor effect on the child who prefers to take part in sedentary activities, while a child who enjoys physical activities runs a greater risk of major changes in self-concept.

Wright also identifies a *status-value* gradient. This relates the person's attributes of self-concept and self-esteem together. Since physical health is invariably a core concept of the individual's self-concept, it necessarily plays a major role in determining self-esteem.

When new information is consistent with the individual's self-concept, the two can be integrated together without problem. Information that is not consistent may be more difficult to deal with. It can be ignored as long as possible. The problem in integrating new inconsistent information is that the existing self-concept determines which aspects of environmental information are attended to. Thus, the person who feels inferior because of a physical illness or disability will expect others to react to such worthlessness, whether or not they do so genuinely. Negative self-concepts therefore become self-perpetuating.

Wright suggests therefore that adjustment to physical disability is dependent on *acceptance* of the disability and appropriate *value changes*. Acceptance amounts to a lack of denial of the disability. When disability occurs, the individual's characteristics most affected are excluded from central aspects of the self-concept. Disadvantages of the disability are thus difficult to overcome. As a result, the individual is unable to come to terms with the disability, and similarly cannot believe that others will accept the condition. In essence, if the individual does not accept the physical disability, it cannot be expected that others will be able to accept it.

At the same time, Wright suggests, the individual must reorganize his or her personal value systems. Physical health and appearance need to be downgraded in value and other attributes found to take their place.

Coping Approaches

Adjustment to physical disorder has also been related to the development of specific coping and defensive strategies. Lipowski (1970) defined coping as all cognitive and motor activities employed by an individual to preserve bodily and physical integrity, the recovery of reversibly impaired function, and compensation for any irreversible impairment. Determinants of coping include *intrapersonal* factors (age, personality, intelligence), *disease-related* factors (severity, chronicity) and *environmental* factors (family communication and interaction). These factors are discussed more fully in Chapter 4.

Similarly, Mattson (1972) argues that coping behaviors included "all the adaptational techniques used by an individual to master a major psychological threat and its attendant negative feelings in order to allow him to achieve personal and social goals" (p. 805). Coping techniques employed by children can be categorized as follows:

1. *Cognitive functions of memory, language and reasoning.* Coping skills based on these processes should enable the child to accept limitations imposed by the illness, assume as much responsibility for his or her own care as possible, and assist (or cooperate) in the medical management of the condition.
2. *Compensatory physical and intellectual activities.* These may develop as new areas of interest and adaptive functioning.
3. *Appropriate release and control of emotions.* The child must learn to express anger and frustration associated with the disease in socially accepted ways and on appropriate occasions.
4. *Withdrawal and demandingness.* On some occasions it may be appropriate for the child to withdraw from such social activity in order to build up strength to combat the disease.
5. *Defensive strategies to manage the anxiety.* A degree of denial of the extent of disability associated with the illness can be useful in enabling the individual to achieve in certain areas.

In combining these two models, Pless and Pinkerton (1975) are primarily concerned with emphasizing that the process of adaptation to illness is not static. Their model is summarized in Figure 1-1. Many of the intrapersonal type of factors described by Lipowski (1970) are dependent on genetic and other familial factors. At the same time, these attributes influence the child's self-concept and coping style. In this way, Pless and Pinkerton argue that assessments of the psychological effects of chronic illness on the child need to take account of the premorbid personality. (While recognizing the logic of this argument, it is not easy to see exactly how this might be done empirically.)

The child's response is also thought to depend on the nature of the illness and the reactions of significant others.

Partly these are reactions to the disorder *per se*, but additionally they are reactions to the behaviour of the child in relation to his illness. As time progresses, successive cycles of these major determinants (of coping and self-concept) will evolve; so that, at any given point, adjustment or

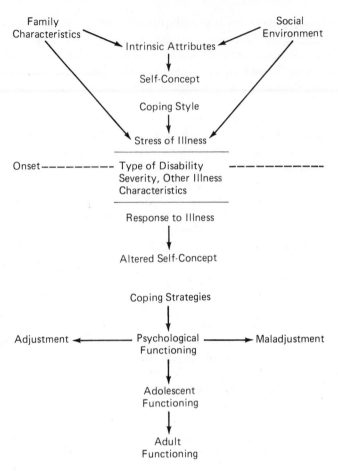

Figure 1-1. An integrated model of adjustment. (Adapted from Pless, I. B. & Pinkerton, P. (1975). *Chronic childhood disorder, promoting patterns of adjustment.* London: Henry Kimpton, p. 25. with permission.)

maladjustment, in terms of psychological functioning, will reflect the net product of earlier cycles. (Pless & Pinkerton, 1975, p. 30)

The practical implications of this model are that the earlier intervention techniques occur, the greater the chance of improving adjustment and preventing maladjustment.

The concepts of adjustment or coping in relation to chronic illness are, in themselves, arbitrary. Coping has been variously viewed as a strategy for dealing with threat (Lazarus, 1966) or problem-solving behaviors to meet the demands of life (Mechanic, 1968). According to Lipowski (1970), chronic illness is seen not only as a severe threat to the individual, but also as an opportunity to develop adaptational behaviors that may result in psychological growth. Mattson (1972) also recognizes the potential opportunity for development that is associated with chronic illness. He defines coping behaviors as those that involve adaptational techniques to master severe stress and allow personal and social goals to be achieved. In the reviews that follow, there is some evidence that any single definition of coping or adjustment is necessarily inappropriate in a developmental context. The process of adjustment to illness by a 3-year-old cannot be assumed to be the same as that made by a 12-year-old. In the following chapters, an attempt will be made to consider how adjustment to illness may vary as a function of a child's level of cognitive development.

The following chapters will present discussions of the degree to which variables such as those previously described have been successful in predicting the child's response to illness. In addition, it will be argued that an understanding of the processes whereby the normal healthy child gains an awareness of concepts of health and illness is basic to understanding the psychology of the sick child. Any comprehensive account of the effects of chronic illness on children must not be limited simply to a description of rates of "maladjustment" in the children or degree of "stress" experienced by the families. As Rutter (1981) has argued previously, such terms have been used so interchangeably that they lack any kind of predictive validity. Many issues of central relevance to the care and understanding of sick children have been essentially neglected or poorly studied. Thus, little attention has been given to the question of what chronically sick children should be told about their condition, or when they should be told. How should we modify accounts of the disease process and treatment for children of different chronological age, personality, or social situation? Even more important, how does knowledge of this kind influence, if at all, the child's acceptance of the condition and adherence to treatment? What aspects of the illness disturb the children; are they bothered about the prognosis for the future or simply worried about explaining school absence to peers?

Similar questions can be posed about parental reactions. The parents' understanding of the disease has implications not only for their own management of the child's disease, but also because they are invariably the child's major source of information. Their misunderstandings and misgivings about the cause of the disease or its treatment are thereby perpetuated. Garson, Benson, Ivler, and Patton, (1978) have listed the many questions that parents of children with congenital heart disease would like to know, but are less frequently told.

While there has been much research focusing on the effects of the disease on the child's development, and separately for the parents on their adjustment and relationships with others, there has been considerably less concern with the dynamics of the parent–child relationship.

However, in coming to terms with the child's illness it is probable that significant changes occur in the parents' immediate expectations of the child and in their hopes for the future. In turn, such changes are likely to have repercussions for both the child's academic and social behaviors.

The main thesis of this book is, then, that understanding the process whereby the normal child gains an awareness of concepts of health and illness is basic to understanding the psychology of the sick child. The study of the chronically sick child needs to encompass a wider range of behaviors than has been customary in the past. For example, research needs to consider the extent of parents' and children's understanding of the disease and its process, and how, if at all, this relates to management of disease and compliance with treatment. In this respect there needs to be some consideration of the type of information that patients and their families would like to have, as well as the information that medical staff feel they ought to have. Much evidence suggests that the two are not the same, and that in fact there may be predictable differences between children of different chronological ages and adults in terms of what they would like to know (cf., Bibace & Walsh, 1981).

This book, then, is not simply a catalog of how chronic illness influences children and their families. There have been many commendable attempts to do this in the past. For example, Katz (1963) has discussed the child's development following hemophilia; Davis (1963), following polio; Goldin, Perry, Margolin, Stotsky, and Foster (1971) and Bagley (1971), following epilepsy; Roskies (1972), following damage resulting from thalidomide treatment; and Schlesinger and Meadow (1972), following deafness. Both Patterson, Denning, and Kutscher (1973) and Burton (1975) have described the effects of cystic fibrosis on children and their families; Garner and Thompson (1974b) and S. B. Johnson (1980), of diabetes; and Schulman and Kupst (1980), Kellerman (1980), and Koocher and O'Malley (1981), of leukemia. There have been somewhat fewer attempts to draw this work together and consider the effects of illness more generally (Grave & Pless, 1974; Lansdown, 1980; McCollum, 1981; Pless & Pinkerton, 1975; Travis, 1976). Briefer summaries are also given by Mattson (1972) and Lavigne and Burns (1981). While much of this work is interesting in itself, it is difficult to see what implications can be drawn for situations involving other illnesses or other patients differing in age, social class, or related variables. In this book some attempt is made to organize reviews of specific illnesses round some common themes. In this way, implications of findings for one disease can be integrated more readily into findings from another.

In most of the literature the emphasis is on the *effect of chronic illness on children and their families*. More recently, it has been recognized that any repercussions of chronic illness are dependent on an individual's response, rather than fashioned by the disease. In all aspects of medicine, including pediatrics, there is a recognition of the fact that success is dependent on the combined resources of physician, child, and family, and that aspects of management need to be negotiated between the three (cf., Strowig, 1982).

For these reasons, the book begins with a description of the development of concepts of health and illness among children. We first trace the development of children's beliefs about the causes and prevention of illness and their definitions of health and behaviors they think important in maintaining health. There is beginning to be considerable evidence that children's beliefs about these issues develop in a systematic, predictable sequence. By acknowledging the existence of this sequence, it should, in theory, be possible to modify information about the cause of their illness and reasons for their treatment to suit the needs of children across a range of ages. At the same time, this research has consistently shown that children's concerns about illness differ from those of adults. For example, children define illness differently from adults (Campbell, 1975) and are more concerned with the social limitations imposed by illness than the physical ramifications (Millstein, Adler, & Irwin, 1981).

Having described in detail the development of the normal child's beliefs about health and illness, we next consider the development of the chronically sick child from a similar point of view. Most sick children spend a proportion of their time in hospital, if not as an inpatient, then at least as a regular outpatient, which is routinely required. Their perceptions of hospitals, nursing staff, and medical treatment may therefore be central in determining their more general adjustment to the disease. In particular, considerable attention is given to reviewing studies in which attempts to prepare children for hospital admission have been made. Such studies are criticized precisely because they fail to take account of differences between adults and children in terms of *what* they would like to know.

There follows a general review of the established literature concerned with the effects of chronic illness on the child and the family in general, but especially the parents, and the siblings. This chapter aims to give a general overview of the field before discussing the effects of some specific illnesses in more detail. Psychological effects of phenyl-ketonuria, diabetes, asthma, and leukemia are considered at length. This is clearly not an exhaustive list of all chronic conditions that might affect children. Diseases involving known involvement of the central nervous system or gross physical handicap have deliberately been excluded. For the moment, the concern is with children who, despite chronic illness, are treated as healthy children and expected to behave as such. Two additional factors have influenced the selection of diseases to be discussed. The first relates to the incidence of the disease among

Table 1-3. Leading Causes of Death Among Children in the United States, 1978

Cause (by Rank)	Incidences (%)
Accidents	47.0
Cancer	10.3
Congenital abnormalities	8.2
Homicide	3.8
Pneumonia and flu	3.2
Heart disease	3.1
Cerebrovascular disease	1.5
Meningitis	1.5
Cerebral palsy	1.3
Cystic fibrosis	1.1
Anemias	.8
Menigoccal infections	.8
Suicide	.8
Epilepsy	.6
Benign neoplasms	.6
All others	.6

Data from "Cancer Statistics, 1982" by E. Silverberg, 1982, *Ca-A Cancer Journal for Clinicians, 32(1)*, p. 30. Copyright 1982 by the American Cancer Society, Inc.

children. Causes of mortality and morbidity according to the 1978 U.S. census (Silverberg, 1982) are given in Table 1-3. After accidents, cancer is the leading cause of death among children, and acute leukemia the most common form of childhood cancer. Partly because leukemia is a highly emotive term and partly because of the lengthy, unpredictable course of treatment, the psychological problems created in caring for these children are considerable. Leukemia is therefore justifiably included both on grounds of prevalence and on grounds of psychological distress involved.

Other diseases have been chosen because they too have aroused considerable research interest in the past. They also clearly involve an interdisciplinary approach to care. Phenylketonuria leads to mental retardation unless treated as soon as possible after birth. Psychologists have been involved in assessing the effectiveness of treatment, that is, checking that the child's intelligence does not deteriorate. Treatment is primarily by diet, and there has been a recent concern with how parents manage to maintain a child on the diet. Parental objections to the diet have led to pressure on pediatricians to relax the diet wherever possible, and again psychologists have been closely involved in monitoring any untoward effects that this may have.

Both diabetes and asthma are relatively common conditions of childhood, and both require long-term treatment and cooperation with physicians. In both cases, it is clear that it is insufficient to inform patients of their treatment and expect them to comply. Instead, efforts to secure the child's cooperation and instill a responsibility for self-care appear essential in the management of these diseases. Once again, the argument is that such a degree of self-involvement in care can only develop where attention is paid to the individual child's cognitive understanding of the illness.

2

Children's Knowledge About Their Bodies and Illness

Development of Children's Ideas About Bodies

> Slugs and snails and puppy-dog tails,
> That's what little boys are made of,
> Sugar and spice and all things nice,
> That's what little girls are made of.
> (Children's nursery rhyme)

Ordinary people have very poor knowledge of the inside of their bodies. While they may be sure that their insides are not as described in the nursery rhyme, there is a great deal of confusion, both among children and adults, as to what the inside of their body is like. Boyle (1970) for example, found that the majority of his adult sample could not correctly locate the stomach, heart, kidney, or liver. Blum (1977) studied undergraduate students and asked them to draw and label internal body organs on an outline diagram. Of those who included a heart, 11% misplaced it. Only a minority drew a liver, and of these 57% misplaced it. A more recent study by Pearson and Dudley (1982) showed that people not only have very poor knowledge about their bodies, but also that what knowledge they have is often erroneous. Eleven of 81 subjects believed that they had two livers, one on each side of the body, and 15 that the gallbladder is located in the pelvic area.

Yet while adults may lack correct information and often be misinformed about their bodies, children, it has been argued, harbor some quaint misconceptions. Very young children can have no way of knowing what might be inside their bodies apart from their knowledge about what they themselves have put there. Hence, the characteristic drawings of the inside of their bodies by young children are often

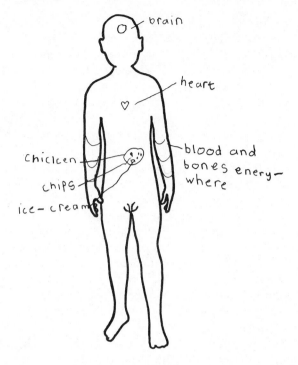

brain

heart

Chicken

chips

ice-cream

blood and bones enery-where

Figure 2-1. Drawing of the inside of the body by a 7-year-old (from Eiser & Patterson, 1983).

liberally decorated with slices of apple pie, chicken, and chips (Figure 2-1).

The study of an individual's knowledge of and attitude toward the body is both a neglected and poorly investigated issue. It is important for two reasons. First, much health education is dependent on an adequate knowledge of anatomy and physiology. In deciding on a health education curriculum appropriate for children of different ages, some account of the probable level of this knowledge needs to be taken. Second, this research has relevance for dealing with chronically sick children. Explanations of illness, its treatment, and consequences should not simply be *précis* versions of medical textbooks, but made appropriate to the child's cognitive status.

The suggestion that these issues have been poorly investigated rests on two grounds. First, there is a general confusion over exactly what is being investigated. There often is a confusion between an individual's factual knowledge of anatomy and more psychological aspects of body image and self-concept. These two components of the problem need to be kept quite distinct. Second, there are methodological problems in the way this research tends to have been conducted. Almost without exception, data have been obtained by asking subjects to draw what is inside their bodies. Such a method does have the advantage of being language free, and therefore it has been assumed that children's drawings will reflect their knowledge and be unaffected by linguistic constraints. By the same token, though, the accuracy with which children are able to draw their bodies will be dependent, in part, on their graphic skills. The task is a difficult one. Aside from general considerations are the major problems of depicting a three-dimensional object in a two-dimensional form (Freeman, 1972). Some authors have therefore attempted to simplify the task by asking children to draw a circle to depict where certain major organs are sited.

Schilder and Wechsler (1935) are to be credited with the first investigation in this area. However, although they claim to have studied 40 children systematically, the data are not presented in such a way that many conclusions can be drawn. The children were aged between 4 and 13 years and were simply asked to name what was inside their bodies. The youngest children consistently believed that food was inside them— not an unreasonable guess as we pointed out earlier. Schilder and Wechsler reported that children over 11 years gave correct answers, although the authors do not elaborate on how complex these answers were.

Tait and Ascher (1955) asked subjects to draw the insides of their bodies on an outline figure. Subjects were both adults and school children (aged between 11 and 13 years). On average, subjects drew and correctly labeled six to nine body parts. The heart was the most popular item. Children tended to emphasize skeletomuscular parts of the body and omitted reproductive organs, while adults included reproductive organs and omitted skeletomuscular systems. A subsample of adult surgical patients drew the organ or system to be operated on with greater than average frequency, suggesting perhaps that an individual's view of the body can be affected by illness status.

Subsequent work moved away from such a psychoanalytic tradition and adopted a more developmental approach. Gellert (1962) studied 96 children, aged between 5 and 17 years. All were hospitalized at the time of testing, for a variety of conditions, both acute and chronic. The children were asked to name the parts of their body and then to draw given organs (e.g., heart, brain, lungs) on an outline figure. They were also asked a number of questions about body parts.

The mean number of body parts correctly drawn increased from 3.3 for the youngest group (aged between 5 and 7 years) to 14.0 for the oldest group (aged 13 to 17 years). Children rarely named or drew reproductive organs. The five most frequently mentioned items across all age groups were bones, blood vessels, heart, blood, and brain. As might be expected, both intuitively and from Tait and Ascher's (1955) study, many children mentioned items associated with illness or surgery

Table 2-1. Percentages of Children Naming the Brain, Bones, and Heart, as Reported in the Literature

Parts Named	Tait & Ascher (1955) (%)	Gellert (1962) (%)	Porter (1974) (%)
Brain	82	39	87
Bones	36	74	93
Heart	64	57	99

(i.e., the appendix was mentioned by 20% of the children and the tonsils by 25%).

These last results suggest the possibility that children's views of their bodies are influenced by temporary phenomena, such as being in the hospital. Perhaps for this reason, a similar study was reported by Porter (1974), in which 144 healthy schoolchildren took part. The children were divided into three age-groups of 6-, 8-, and 10-year-olds. Testing was carried out in the classroom, with outline figures being distributed, and the children were asked to draw what was inside them. Porter's main finding was that children of all ages were able to name more body parts than had been reported in previous studies (see Table 2-1).

In other ways, too, Porter was impressed with children's level of knowledge. "Some surprisingly detailed and intricate parts of the inside of the body were named by the subjects, particularly the fifth-graders: adenoids, "air-bags," bone marrow, cerebellum, cerebrum, cortex, eustacian tube, eye-socket, "fatty-layer," "growth plate," optic nerve, pancreas, pores, schlera, tooth-root" (1974, p. 38)—impressive indeed. Porter also noted that organs tended to be drawn with accuracy and were relatively proportionate. Correct medical terms were used with very little slang or lay terms, even among the 6-year-olds. No consistent sex differences were found.

In discussing the results, Porter (1974) draws implications for health education, emphasizing the need not to talk down to children, whose knowledge is possibly greater than adults generally think. However, there is one methodological flow in all this: Porter admits that some cheating may have occurred in the classroom. If it did, this may have given a false impression of the children's knowledge.

These preliminary attempts to record how children view the insides of their bodies may be interesting, but do not go much beyond a simple listing of body parts known to children at different ages. That children's knowledge increases with age is hardly surprising. Of potentially greater interest may be questions related to how such knowledge is acquired. For example, why does the child's knowledge tend to proceed in a given order? Why do children first gain knowledge about the heart, to be followed by knowledge about the brain and stomach, and only later about the lungs? At the same time, for the average child and adult too, knowledge about organs such as the kidneys, liver, and bladder is usually minimal. An attempt to organize previous findings according to a theoretical framework that might also predict some answers to these questions of ordering was proposed by Crider (1981).

Crider (1981) interviewed 21 children between the ages of 6 and 12 years. Each child was asked to name what was inside the body, draw it, and then locate different organs on a human figure drawing provided by the examiner. The child was also asked to describe the function of different body organs, and to describe what happens to food eaten and air breathed. Based on these data (which are not described in detail), Crider hypothesized that the child's knowledge of the body progresses through a systematic and predictable sequence. Thus, during the *preoperational* phase, the child perceives body functioning in a relatively global way, with no clear distinction between internal and external. Hence, the young child shows a tendency to include items of food in drawings of the body. At this stage, too, functions are perceived in terms of purpose or final causes, for example, that lungs are for breathing.

During the *concrete operational* phase, the child becomes able to differentiate structures and their function. At this stage, functions are perceived in terms of coordinated movements in space and time, relating different perceived states to one another. For example, muscles are in the leg to help it bend; the child perceives the leg bending and attributes the cause of this movement to the muscles. Finally, at a *formal operational* stage, the child is able to posit hypothetical transformations to account for body functioning. At this stage, too, functions are hierarchically orgaized in terms of organs, systems, and the interdependence of systems.

This theory, though impressive on first reading, is rather disappointing. It is very difficult to translate into empirical terms; neither does it generate any new hypotheses about how the child acquires knowledge of the body. Indeed, even Crider (1981) seemed disinclined to pursue the ideas further. Instead, she chose to emphasize the need to distinguish between cognitive and affective components of individual's body knowledge.

This distinction between cognitive and affective components of an individual's body knowledge is especially critical in dealing with maladjusted children or the chronically sick. Unfortunately it is in just such studies of the chronically sick that most confusion has occurred. Shontz (1971) has pointed out that there is generally a failure to distinguish between the effects of an individual's body image and the direct effects of the physical disorder, self-concept, and social responses to changes in physique. Despite these criticisms, it has been reported that some changes in body knowledge or image occur among children undergoing surgery (Gellert, 1962), children with heart disease (Auer, Senturia, & Shopper, 1971; Green & Levitt, 1962), cystic fibrosis (Boyle, di Sant' Agnese, Sack, Millican, & Kukzycki, 1976), and diabetes (Eiser, Patterson, & Tripp, 1984a; Kaufman & Hersher, 1971).

In the study by Green and Levitt (1962), drawings of the body made by 25 children with heart disease were compared with those of 25 healthy children. Those with heart disease drew smaller and less well-developed bodies than the healthy children. Green and Levitt suggested that this might indicate that children with heart disease have a "constricted" self-image, but these interpretations are complicated by the fact that the children genuinely were physically smaller than their healthy counterparts. Auer et al. (1971) noted that children with heart disease were more likely to include a heart on diagrams of the body than healthy children. In addition, those who had undergone surgery were more likely to draw bones than children who had not been treated in this way.

Two separate studies concerned with children with diabetes have shown that some distortions in body knowledge and attitudes exist, although there is some discrepancy as to the degree of distortion. Kaufman and Hersher (1971) concluded that severe distortions in body image occur among diabetic children. Some patients apparently believed that their pancreas was completely missing, others that they had an enormous stomach, since they had to eat so much food. Eiser, Patterson, and Tripp (1984a) did not find evidence of such dramatic changes in body knowledge, but did conclude that diabetes affects the child's attitude toward the body. Both these studies are considered in greater detail in Chapter 6.

Finally, Boyle et al. (1976) investigated knowledge of the body among a group of children with cystic fibrosis. This disease might be expected to influence a child's general body image to a significant degree. Affected children tend to be smaller and less well-developed than their peers and are required to undergo regular physiotherapy. The burdens faced by families with a child with cystic fibrosis are described sympathetically by Burton (1975). In the study by Boyle et al. (1976), 27 patients between the ages of 13 and 30 years were interviewed, as were their mothers. Of particular relevance were data obtained about the patients' attitudes toward their bodies. All apparently expressed dissatisfaction with their bodies. On the whole, patients were skilled at using clothing and hairstyles to disguise their thinness, but a few had given up. One patient reportedly refused to take baths, she so disliked the look of her body. Seventeen of the 27 patients drew very immature figure drawings showing "striking denial of sexual differences." In contrast, a few of the patients drew exaggeratedly developed "Super-man" bodies. It was clear that none of the subjects felt happy about their body-shape.

There is a general assumption that a "healthy" attitude to the body is associated with a good adjustment to the disease (Lavigne & Burns, 1981). However, there is little empirical work directed at this question. Future studies need to distinguish clearly between affective and cognitive components of a child's body image, and also to link precisely the mechanisms whereby self-image is indicative of more general attitudes to disease.

In addition, there is a need to devise new research methods. Investigators have relied heavily on subjects' drawings of their bodies, yet this method may mask related misconceptions regarding body functions. Patients' beliefs about why people need to eat or breathe, for example, may be as revealing as the more simple knowledge relating to position of the stomach or lungs. A study by Johnson and Wellman (1982) is relevant here.

Johnson and Wellman (1982) investigated children's concepts of the mind and brain. In one study reported, three groups of children (aged 5–6 years, 8–9 years, and 10–11 years) and a group of adults were studied. Subjects were asked to make judgments as to whether the brain was involved in a large number of activities. Children were also asked to locate the brain and describe what it did.

Johnson and Wellman found that all the children were able to locate their brain, and all but one kindergarten child gave a reasonable account of the function of the brain. Children of all ages and adults were consistent in reporting that the brain was needed for mental acts. Other categories of explanation showed age-related changes. Compared with other age-groups for example, 6-year-olds tended to deny that the brain was involved in the senses or simple motor behavior. Children of all ages tended not to report that the brain was involved in involuntary movements, while adults did. The authors concluded that very young children simply regard the brain as involved with mental-intellectual acts. They did not think that the brain was involved in motor tasks, believing that only peripheral body parts were involved (e.g., your feet can walk for you). Both the 8- and 10-year-old children showed a more comprehensive view of brain function, but only the adults included the execution of sensory-motor acts or involuntary movements as under the control of the brain.

Similar conclusions were reached by Eiser and Patterson (1983). As part of a larger study into knowledge of the body, children aged between 6 and 11 years were asked which parts were involved in eating and swimming. The youngest children insisted that the mouth and teeth alone were involved in eating. Older children included the stomach, and later still (11 years) included organs such as the bladder involved in removing waste food. They also mentioned that food was transformed and circulated round the body as blood. Similarly, the 6-year-olds reported that only the arms and legs were needed for swimming. On further questioning, 6-year-olds suggested that the bones made the arms and legs move. Only among 9-year-olds did a proportion of children mention the role of the lungs in swimming or brain in controlling movements. Indeed, only 54% of 12-year-olds thought to mention that the brain was involved in swimming.

Development of Children's Ideas About Illness

Early work concerned with children's understanding of the cause of illness was consistent in concluding that children tended to blame themselves for illness, and view the illness and its treatment as a form of punishment (Langford, 1948; Richter, 1943). Perhaps we should not be surprised at this. In many cases of illness there are no simple explanations, so it is reasonable to look for an explanation in terms of some aspect of personal behavior. Parents faced with a diagnosis of chronic or fatal disease in their child may also look for an explanation in terms of some action of their own (Comaroff & Maguire, 1981). A quotation from Langford (1948) shows how such beliefs may develop and that certain naive theories are communicated directly to children by parents.

> Parental admonitions intensify any latent fear that the child may have that his illness comes as a punishment. Colds come because the child disobeys and does not wear his rubbers. A leg is broken because the child does not heed his mother's cautioning advice not to roller skate in the street. Upset stomach could be avoided if the child would only eat what he is supposed to. Eyes are ruined by fine print or reading in poor light or from too assiduous attention to the comics. The warnings about what will happen are often supplemented with an "I told you so" when something does happen to the child. These are common statements by almost all parents and contribute to the child's idea that when he is sick he is being punished. The all too common practice of threatening the child with the doctor or an operation if he continues to be bad (which to many parents means disobedience) lends further reality to the child's fears when he becomes sick and he is taken for medical advice. (p. 244)

Some empirical studies have provided support for the view that children may interpret illness as a form of punishment. Brodie (1974) reported that 25% of a sample of children believed that "boys and girls who misbehave get sick more often that those who are good" (p. 1157). Cook (1975) also reported that children's spontaneous accounts of illness involved similar moral overtones.

It is apparent that while children may well believe that illness results from misbehavior, they also hold other beliefs about illness causation. A second commonly held view is that illness is caused by germs (Palmer & Lewis, 1975; Perrin & Gerrity, 1979).

Kister and Patterson (1980) studied children's use of contagion and immanent justice (the degree to which undesirable outcomes were directly the result of misdemeanour) in explaining illness. Fifteen children at each of four age-levels were studied. Children were asked a series of questions about (1) a contagious illness (a cold), (2) a noncontagious illness (toothache), and (3) a common accident (scraped knee). Younger children were more likely than older children to use an explanation involving contagion for both contagious and noncontagious illness and accidents. In addition, they did not understand the effect of distance between people influencing the probability of transmitting contagious disease. Young children were more likely to invoke immanent justice as an explanation for all events. At the same time, all the children were more likely to invoke immanent justice explanations for illness rather than accident. A child's tendency to offer immanent justice explanations was inversely related to the level of understanding of the rational causes of illness.

In their earlier review, Bibace and Walsh (1981) concluded that explanations of illness offered by younger children differed from those offered by older children in the following ways. Younger children naturally offered less complex explanations (Natapoff, 1978; Perrin & Gerrity, 1979) and relied less on internal body cues to indicate the presence of illness (Natapoff, 1978; Neuhauser, Amsterdam, Hines, & Steward, 1978). In contrast, older children evidenced more realism (Palmer & Lewis, 1975), more restricted definitions of specific illness (Campbell, 1975), greater generalization based on principle, and a more organized description of process and cause (Perrin & Gerrity, 1979). They also employed more categories to define health and illness than the younger children (Caradang, Folkins, Hines, & Steward, 1979; Natapoff, 1978).

For the purpose of this review, two distinct approaches to studying the child's ideas about causation of illness will be identified. The first puts a sociological emphasis on the child's reasoning (Campbell, 1975); the second adopts a purely cognitive approach (Bibace & Walsh, 1981).

Sociological Approaches

Campbell (1975) has drawn on well-established findings that an individual's definitions of health and illness and illness-related behavior are socially and culturally determined (Mishler, et al., 1981). Children must learn sick-role behavior and related health beliefs from adults and especially from the mother. Campbell identified two processes in the acquisition of adult concepts: (1) *patterned similarity*, which is defined as an emerging consensus on illness definitions with the child's definitions becoming more like adults with age, and (2) *developmental changes in illness concepts*.

Table 2-2. Coding Categories Used to Describe Childrens' Definitions of Illness (Campbell, 1975)

Theme of Coding Category	Example of Responses
1. Nonlocalized, nonspecific feeling state	"Feeling bad," "not right"
2. Nonlocalized, specific feeling state	"Pain," "soreness," "dizzy"
3. Localized and specified somatic feelings	"Head throbs," "stomach hurts"
4. Visible external signs	"Swollen joints," "spitting up stuff"
5. Objective signs not immediately visible	"Hot forehead," "sugar in urine"
6. Disease concept or specific diagnosis	"Appendicitis," "chicken-pox"
7. Mood motivational, attitudinal states	"Grouchy," "irritable," "lazy"
8. Increase in sick role behavior	"Want to lie down," "tell mother I'm sick," "go to bed"
9. Altered conventional role	"Let work go," "stay home from school," "don't play"
10. Behavior or intention of others	"Mother gives me medicine," "doctor gives me shot"
11. Explicit restriction of illness concept	"If I just have a cold, I'm not sick"

Note. From "Illness is a point of view: The development of children's concepts of illness" by J. D. Campbell, 1975, *Child Development, 46*(1). reprinted by permission of the Society for Research in Child Development, University of Chicago Press.

In the study by Campbell (1975) 264 children aged between 6 and 12 years and their mothers were questioned about their definitions of illness. All the children were short-stay (less than 5 days) hospitalized patients (and were chosen so that illness was salient to the children at the time). Campbell was able to categorize children's responses into 11 categories (see Table 2-2). With increasing age of the child, children's definitions became closer to those given by mothers. In addition, Campbell identified a *definitional sophistication.* Younger children defined illness in terms of feeling states. With age, there was an increase in precision of definition. This included specific diagnosis and qualifications stating what illness was not. While the work by Campbell suggests that a child's mother is one influence on the development of views of illness, it is clear that the mother is not the only influence. This preliminary study by Campbell does not actually offer any alternative explanations as to the source of influence on the child's development. Neither did it investigate how the child's own history of illness affects definitions.

Table 2-3. Thematic Profiles in Adolescents, Children, and Adults (from Millstein, Adler, & Irwin, 1981)

Definitional Theme	Adolescents ($n = 77$) (%)	Adults ($n = 263$) (%)	Children $n = 262$) (%)
1	39.0	52.1	60.3
2	51.9	44.5	36.6
3	42.9	25.1	46.2
4	15.6	8.0	11.5
5	5.2	27.8	12.6
6	10.4	28.1	9.5
7	9.1	27.0	11.8
8	9.1	28.5	13.0
9	28.6	42.6	10.7
10	2.6	14.8	8.8
11	0.0	24.0	2.3

Note: Theme numbers correspond to entries in Table 2-2, under Theme of coding category.
Note. From Millstein, Adler & Irwin, 1981. Copyright American Academy of Pediatrics 1981.

Millstein, Adler, and Irwin (1981) extended Campbell's study by investigating concepts of illness among adolescents. Seventy-seven adolescents aged between 11 and 15 years were included. One of the main aims of the study was to investigate more fully any developmental sequence in the type of definitions of illness given, as described in the preliminary study by Campbell (1975). The results are shown in Table 2-3, and do not obviously fit the pattern hypothesized by Campbell. Only one "theme" showed a clearly age-related shift. Definitions involving an "inability to participate in usual activities" were included by only 10.7% of children, 28.6% of adolescents, and 42.5% of adults. Campbell also suggested that themes involving disease states increased with age, but there was in fact little difference between adolescents and children in their use of this definition (10.4% and 9.5%, respectively, compared with 28.1% for adults). Other themes that were expected to increase with age did not show the predicted trend. This applies to themes of "objective signs," "attitude" or "mood" states, and "altered conventional role."

It is unfortunate that the results of this study are so confusing. Millstein et al. (1981) were forced to speculate about the lack of predicted results and suggest that the children studied were of poor intellect. One is therefore left wondering as to whether clear developmental shifts might have been obtained with other samples. There would seem to be a need to replicate this study using tighter methodological criteria. Millstein et al. simply questioned adolescents and borrowed data reported by Campbell for children and adults. Any number of differences in populations or interviewers style might therefore account for these results.

Notwithstanding these criticisms, Millstein et al. do make some very sensible recommendations. They conclude:

> Lay definitions of illness, including those of adolescents, center around symptoms and alterations in the ability to participate in everyday activities. Relatively few children or adolescents define illness in terms of diagnosis. Although most patients seeking health care have somatic complaints, our data suggest that the clinician who communicates with the adolescent patient solely in terms of signs, symptoms, and disease may be neglecting other avenues of communication that are salient to the patient. Discussing the concerns of adolescents that relate to changes in social functioning associated with illness may be a more effective mode of communication. (1981, p. 838)

Cognitive-Developmental Approaches

The main proponents of this approach have been Bibace and Walsh (1980, 1981). They argue that children's concepts of illness will parallel the findings of Piaget (1930) and Werner (1948) regarding the onto-genesis of causal reasoning. It is assumed that "variation in degree of differentiation between the self and the other will manifest itself in significant differences in children's conceptions of health and illness" (Bibace & Walsh, 1980, p. 912).

Bibace and Walsh (1980) interviewed three groups of children. There were 24 children at three age-levels, 4-, 7-, and 11-year-olds. A "concept of illness protocol" was developed and is shown in Table 2-4. Children's responses were then coded according to the three major types of explanation consistent with Piaget's (Piaget, 1930) stages of cognitive development—prelogical, concrete logical, and formal logi-cal. Within each of these categories, two subtypes of explanation were also made. In addition, a few of the youngest children were apparently unable to comprehend the question at all, and were placed in an "incomprehension" category.

Prelogical explanations

Children between the ages of 2 and 6 years offering prelogical explanations of illness appeared excessively swayed by the immediacy of some aspects of their perceptual experiences. The most develop-mentally immature explanation of illness was described as *phenomenism*. Bibace and Walsh characterized this phase as when the cause of illness is seen to be an external concrete phenomenon that may occur with the illness but is spatially and temporally remote. Children are unable to

Table 2-4. Concept of Illness Protocol (Bibace & Walsh, 1980)

Questions Asked of Children

1. What does it mean to be healthy?
2. Do you remember anyone who was not healthy? What was wrong? How did he get sick? How did he get better?
3. Were you ever sick? How did you get sick? How did you get better?
4. What is the worst sickness to have? Why? What is the best sickness to have? Why?
5. What happens to people when they are sick?
6. What is a cold? How do people get colds? Where do colds come from? What makes colds go away?
7. What are the measles? How do people get measles? What makes measles get better?
8. What is a heart attack? Why do people get heart attacks?
9. What is cancer?
10. What is a head-ache? Why do people get head-aches?
11. Have you ever had a pain? Where? What is pain? Why does it come?
12. What are germs? What do they look like? Can you draw germs? Where do they come from?

Note. From Bibace & Walsh, 1980. Copyright American Academy of Pediatrics, 1980.

offer explanations as to how these events cause illness. The following examples are quoted: "How do people get colds? 'From trees.' How do people get measles? 'From God.' How does God give people measles? 'God does it in the sky' " (1981, p. 36).

However, the most common explanation of illness offered by the child in the prelogical stage of thought is *contagion*. The cause of illness is believed to be in objects or people near but not touching the child. The link between the two maybe in terms of proximity or "magic." *Examples*: "How do people get colds? 'From outside.' How do they get them from outside? 'They just do that's all.' They come when someone else gets near you.' How? 'I don't know—by magic I think' . . . How do people get colds? 'When someone else gets near them' " (Bibace & Walsh, 1981, p. 36).

Concrete-logical explanations

Laurendeau and Pinard (1962) describe the major changes in the thinking of the 7- to 10-year-old child to be due to the increase in ability to differentiate between self and other. The child is clearly able to distinguish between what is internal and external to the self.

Younger children in this stage offer explanations of illness in terms of *contamination*. The child distinguishes between the cause of illness and how it is effective. The cause may be viewed as a person, object, or action outside the child that has a harmful potential for the body. Illness is contracted through the child's body physically contacting the person or object or through the child physically engaging in the action and becoming contaminated. *Examples*: "What is a cold? 'It's like in the wintertime.' How do people get them? 'You're outside without a hat and you start sneezing. Your head would get cold—the cold would touch it— and then it would go all over your body' " (Bibace & Walsh, 1981, p. 36).

A more mature explanation is described as *internalization*. Illness is perceived to be located within the body, but the cause may still be external. This external cause is linked to the internal effect of illness through a process of internalization, for example, swallowing or inhaling. Illness is still, however, described in vague and nonspecific terms, showing the child's confusion about internal organs and their function.

Formal-logical explanations

Bibace and Walsh identify two substages of formal logical thought with regard to the causes of illness, *psychological* and *psychophysiological*. Both are characterized by a clear differentation between the self and other. The source of illness is perceived to be located within the body even though an external agent is seen as the ultimate cause.

Younger children, offering a *physiological* explanation of illness, suggest that the source and nature of illness lie in specific internal physiological structures and functions. The cause is often described as the nonfunctioning or malfunctioning of an internal organ or process.

Finally, Bibace and Walsh (1981) identified the most mature conceptions of illness to be represented by *psychophysiological* explanations. Illness is still described in terms of internal physiological processes, but the child entertains the probability of an alternative, usually psychological cause of the illness. The child becomes aware that an individual's thoughts or feelings can affect the way the body functions.

As would be predicted from a cognitive developmental framework, the frequency with which children used these explanations varied as a function of age. Among 4-year-olds, 54% gave contagion explanations and 38% contamination explanations. Among 7-year-olds, 63% gave contamination and 29% internalization explanations. Among 11-year-olds, explanations were predominantly of the internalization (54%) or physiological (34%) categories.

A very similar approach to that of Bibace and Walsh (1980, 1981) was reported by Perrin and Gerrity (1981). Again children were asked a series of questions about the causes and prevention of different illnesses. Responses were categorized into one of six categories, and Perrin and Gerrity again felt that these were comparable to the stages of cognitive development defined by Piaget (1930). In addition to the questions about illness causation, children also attempted more conventional tests of conservation and transformations. These data showed that the child's understanding of illness causation lagged behind understanding of physical concepts.

Development of Sick Children's Ideas About Illness

In their conclusions, Perrin and Gerrity (1981) state that "the value of improved understanding of the processes of illness is not known. One may speculate that it could result in more sophisticated self-care and preventive health decisions, better compliance with medical care regimes, and more appropriate medical care and medication utilization" (p. 848). Empirical support for these speculations is not yet forthcoming.

Even so, the question of how illness experience might influence the normal process of acquisition of illness concepts is intriguing. Early work tended to imply that the sick child's views on illness causation developed similarly to those of the healthy child. Thus, there are several studies emphasizing that sick children perceive illness as a form of punishment (Beverley, 1936; Brazelton, 1953; Dubo, 1950; Peters, 1975; Richter, 1943).

It is possible that these conclusions were in part due to the methodological techniques used to elicit the data. Often projective techniques were employed. In a study by Schechter (1961) for example, it was reported that "close" questioning consistently uncovered the idea that illness was a punishment for misdemeanor. Whether "close" questioning enables the investigator to get at the child's deep-seated beliefs or reduces the child to saying what the investigator wants to hear is very much dependent on one's point of view.

Two more recent studies (Brewster, 1982; Simeonsson, Buckley, & Monson, 1979) investigated illness concepts in sick children. Although the authors did not compare the sick with a healthy group, they did suggest that the sorts of ideas expressed by sick children are similar to those reported for healthy children in other studies. Thus, the authors suggest that the development of the sick child's ideas is not qualitatively different from that of the healthy child, but they do not provide any information as to whether this development is more or less mature.

Simeonsson et al. (1979) studied 60 hospitalized children, aged 5, 7, and 9 years. The children were asked six questions:

How can children keep from getting sick?
What does medicine do?
How do children get sick?
How do children get stomach-aches?

How do children get bumps or spots?
When children are sick, how do they get better again? (p. 78)

Responses were scored into three categories. The first stage was described as "global" or "undifferentiated," often reflecting magical or superstitious ideas. For example, one girl responded to the question about how children get sick by answering "when you kiss old people and women."

The second stage reflected more concrete and specific ideas. The cause of illness was often associated with the violation of rules. Although the children were aware of some specific actions that caused illness they did not know of any generalized principle. For example, illness was attributed to peanuts going in the wrong pipe, taking medicine you're not supposed to, or eating poison. At the third stage, children showed an awareness of a generalized principle, for example, that illnesses were caused by catching germs from other people and could be alleviated by taking medicines. Simeonson et al. (1979) reported an age-related shift in children's responses, and suggested that improved communication between doctor and child could only be effected by greater awareness of the uniqueness of children's thought.

Brewster (1982) similarly identified three stages in children's cognitions about illness. She studied 50 chronically ill, hospitalized children, aged between 5 and 12 years. She found that most children less than 7 years of age believed that illness was the result of human action, often associated with wrongdoing. Children aged between 7 and 10 years believed that illness was caused by germs. It was not until reaching the age of 11 years that children acknowledged that there could be more than one cause for illness and that the process of becoming ill was the result of an interaction between several factors, including the body's own defence mechanisms and the infection.

Beales, Holt, Keen, and Mellor (1983) interviewed 75 patients with juvenile chronic arthritis about their beliefs about their illness and effectiveness of medical treatment. The patients were divided into two groups; those between 7 and 11 years, and those between 12 and 17 years. Children were first asked what they imagined their arthritis to be, how it affected their body and made the body different from a healthy body. Responses to this question were divided as follows: "subjective feeling ('it makes me feel ill,' 'it makes my finger ache') . . . surface appearance ('it makes my knee look red and swollen') . . . motor ability ('I can't move my neck properly' 'it stops my finger bending') . . . internal pathology ('it damages my bones' 'it fills my joints with blood')" (Beales et al., 1983, p. 482).

Children were then asked to draw what they imagined their affected joints looked like and to describe them. Finally, children were asked about therapy and to explain what the purpose of different medical therapies were. In addition, a fixed-choice questionnaire about the perceived value of treatments was administered.

Beales et al. (1983) noted fundamental differences beween the two age-groups in terms of their beliefs about their illness. The younger children tended to see the illness in terms of concrete signs. They defined arthritis in terms of its effect on their bodies; that it made their knees ache or their finger sore. Beales et al. noted that for the majority of 7- to 11-year-old children, these signs of the illness constituted an adequate explanation of the disease itself. Most 12- to 17-year-olds recognized that these outward signs were the consequences of an internal pathology; their explanations of the disease still tended to be limited, however, focusing on internal damage of bones and blood, with little mention of other tissues. The children's knowledge tended to be oversimplified or exaggerated, resulting in an imagined pathology that was often more severe than was the case.

Beales et al. (1983) noted that younger groups of children had difficulty drawing the insides of affected joints, and were more likely to draw the outside with the joint red and swollen. Older children were more able to draw the "insides," and tended to depict these in terms of damage to bones and blood vessels. Many of these older children registered distaste as soon as they had drawn their bodies.

It is apparent from this study that younger children's misconceptions about the disease process and its effects on their body might lead to conflict in their accepting much of the prescribed treatment. If findings such as these can be replicated, there can surely be no finer argument for better preparation and information about disease to be made available for the young chronically sick child. Beales et al. (1983) conclude that children of different ages require qualitatively different kinds of explanations. While children of 12 years or more can often cope with a medically oriented description of their disease, younger children are more likely to benefit from descriptions that make use of "specific analogies" drawn from their immediate experiences. Thus, blood vessels can be likened to pipelines and nerves to electric wiring. It is suggested that disease activity can be described in military terms: In the case of juvenile arthritis, the explanation might be that the body's defending forces are unable to identify the enemy and have turned on their own side in error.

The results of all these studies suggest that sick children share a similar belief system about illness causation compared with healthy children. None of these studies, however, provide any direct comparison of sick and healthy children. Such a design is essential if we are to understand the processes whereby these concepts are attained. On both intuitive and theoretical grounds, it could be predicted that the experience of chronic illness would influence a child's thinking about illness in general. It is less obvious, however, whether this experience would act to speed the child's cognitions about illness, or retard them.

Piaget (1962) argued that development proceeds at a variable rate depending on both the child's experience with the phenomenon and its associated affect. This assumption might lead us to predict that, because of their increased experience with illness, sick children would have more developed concepts of illness than healthy peers. In fact, the little evidence available does not support this view (Cook, 1975). Indirect evidence comes from a study by Caradang et al. (1979), in which it was found that children with diabetic siblings had less mature concepts of illness than children with healthy siblings. These data support the hypotheses of Bibace and Walsh (1981) that the "experience of illness has such overwhelming emotional concomitants that the level of conceptualization with respect to the illness is inhibited or regressed" (p. 45).

Studies in which sick children have been directly compared with healthy children have highlighted some qualitative differences in reasoning between the two groups. Lynn, Glaser, and Harrison (1962), for example, compared 25 children with rheumatism with healthy controls. Those with rheumatism were significantly more likely to believe that illness was caused by germs, eating dirt or poison, and their own carelessness. Healthy children tended to believe that illness was caused by the elements (i.e., staying out in the cold or wet). Myers-Vando, Steward, Folkins, and Hines (1979) compared adolescents with chronic cardiac disease with healthy controls, and reported that those with chronic illness showed less mature reasoning.

More recently, Eiser, Patterson, and Tripp (1984b) compared 57 children with diabetes with a matched group of healthy children. Subjects were asked a wide range of questions about both health and illness. There were some differences between the two groups in their knowledge of oral hygiene, diet, and nutrition. The groups did not differ in their knowledge of the cause of a variety of illnesses, apart from an expected greater knowledge by diabetics about the cause of diabetes. The groups did not differ significantly either in their definition of "health" although normal children were more likely than diabetics to define health as "not being ill" or "body working properly." Eiser et al. (1984b) concluded that illness was not likely to influence a child's concepts of illness in any simple way. Rather, it was clear that whether or not the sick children appeared to know more or less than the healthy children about some aspects of illness was as dependent on the child's age as on the illness. They point to the need to consider variations in the demands of the illness when predicting how chronic illness affects the child's cognitions.

Most work concerned with the child's understanding of illness has focused on the healthy child's beliefs, or at most, the beliefs of children hospitalized for short periods. While this approach has some advantages, it must be apparent that the real value of this work lies in its ability to make valid recommendations for dealing with the chronically sick. The irony of the situation was summarized by Blos (1978). Most of his comments are still valid.

> It is interesting to note that no study examining the ill child's concepts of health was found. It may be presumed that health professionals, parents and ill children believe health to be so obvious in the face of disease and illness that it does not deserve study. Yet it would be of interest to see if concepts of health and the terms in which they are defined would vary with the severity of illness, chronicity, or residual defect experience. Would we see a conceptual regression, an idealization or some other kind of distortion? This information would seem to be of use in understanding children with long-term illness or permanent handicap, since by helping such children correct distortion, some disappointment might be prevented. (p. 8.)

Development of Children's Ideas About Health

Researchers in this tradition have focused on when, in terms of chronological age, children develop an awareness of concepts of health, and how this awareness changes throughout life. Natapoff (1978) suggests that much of the failure of traditional health education for children can be attributed to a failure to account for differences between adults and children in their cognitive representations of health concepts. Developmental changes in definition of health concepts have been noted by Rashkis (1965), Byler and Lewis (1969), Natapoff (1978), and Eiser, Patterson, and Eiser (1983).

Rashkis (1965) studied the development of the child's view of health by investigating 54 healthy children, aged between 4 and 9 years. He argued that children recognize the limitations of their ability to keep themselves well and are aware of vulnerability to illness. Eating is seen as important in fostering health and appears to figure significantly in the children's ways of coping with the potential threat of illness.

Byler and Lewis (1969) surveyed 5000 children and reported age-related shifts in children's qualitative definitions of health. Third-graders defined health in a variety of ways having to do with behavior and appearance: "Doesn't play with matches"; "Lifts weights"; "Isn't too fat or too skinny" "Combs her hair"; "Smells clean." Fourth-graders responded with greater detail; for example, "is physically fit"; "Does certain amount of walking and running and does exercise"; "Eats everything he should, the right vegetables, not too much fattening food or candy, eats well-balanced diet"; "Keeps clean, washes hands and face before meals, takes a bath every night or so, brushes his teeth, doesn't live in dirty surroundings".

Similar data were presented somewhat more systematically by Natapoff (1978). She studied ninety-one 6-year-olds, eighty-nine 9-year-olds, and eighty-four 12-year-olds. Responses to the question of "What does it feel like to be healthy?" could be grouped into eight categories: feel good (67%), do wanted things (61%), not sick (48%), food (44%), exercise (31%), clean (27%), happy (24%), strong body (23%). With age, children mentioned a greater number of categories. An average of five categories were mentioned by the 6-year-olds, eight by the 9-year-olds and nine by the 12-year-olds. Natapoff further noted that older children were more likely to express doubts about their replies, and acknowledge that the word was difficult to define. Children were also asked "How can you tell when a family member is healthy?" Six-year-olds tended to rely on perceptual data to determine another's health, while even the 12-year-olds found this question difficult.

Eiser et al. (1983) investigated children's ideas of health, illness, and illness prevention. Twenty children at each of four age levels were studied, 6, 8, 9, and 11 years. For all ages combined, children were most likely to define health in terms of taking exercise and being energetic (75%) and eating good food (40%). With increasing age, children defined health as "not being ill" (10%, 35%, 10%, 45%, of the respective age-groups), eating good food (10%, 45%, 45%, 60%, respectively), taking exercise (0%, 55%, 70%, 65%, respectively), and being strong, fit, or full of energy (10%, 20%, 65%, 70%, respectively). Some of the older children stated that being healthy involved an increased resistance to infection (0%, 0%, 5%, 5%, respectively). "Not smoking" was also mentioned by some (5%, 0%, 10%, 5%, respectively).

Children's views on health were further investigated by Gochman (1971) and Gochman, Bagramian, and Sheiham (1972), who argued that from quite young ages, children develop consistent personality differences in their beliefs about their own vulnerability to health problems. Children's perceived vulnerability was investigated by asking them to rate on a 7-point scale "How likely are you to catch a cold during this next year?" The topics included were a bad accident, rash, fever, sore throat, flu, toothache, cold, missing a week off school because of sickness, upset stomach, cutting a finger accidentally, bad headache, poison ivy, sinus trouble, being stung by a bee, and having a cavity. Gochman et al. (1972) reported that at 7 years of age, the children showed a consistent hierarchical pattern of perceived vulnerability to illness. Children's expectations about dental problems acquired consistency earlier than nondental problems. Girls had higher expectancies of health problems than boys, and older children of both sexes had higher levels than 7-year-old girls.

Gochman (1971) attempted to describe how realistic children's estimates of health expectancies were. One year after collection of the data, parents were asked how many days of school were missed for illness. There was no correlation between the number of days of school missed and the child's perceived vulnerability to illness. (Perhaps this result needs to be viewed with caution. The sample size was relatively small, $N = 108$. It is doubtful how accurate parents' recall of absence could be after a 1-year interval; there seems little reason why school records themselves could not have been used.) Finally, Gochman (1971) noted that "health" was not a highly salient issue for these children. He speculates that the concept of health is of little value either to children or to the adults they become; health education is not generally effective simply because health is such a nonsalient issue. This conclusion seems rather unwarranted, however, given the methods by which the data were collected. The "salience" of health was measured as follows: Children were shown a series of pictures that could have some potential for eliciting health-related responses (e.g., children playing near rubbish, a mother and child in front of a medicine cabinet). Children were asked to describe what was going on in each picture. The degree to which the child introduced health topics into the story was taken as indicative of an individual health salience. Perhaps it should not be surprising that such indirect, paper-and-pencil techniques do not suggest that children are overly aware of health issues. It is possible that it is not a lack of interest in health that these studies indicate, but a lack of interest in the methods used. Where children are given greater freedom to define health in their own way, they appear highly interested in health and motivated to learn more (Smith, 1981).

The role of the mother in shaping the child's concepts of health has been documented in some research by Mechanic (1964). He studied 350 children and their mothers living in Wisconsin. The children were divided into two age-groups, 9–10 years and 13–14 years. Mothers were interviewed regarding their attitudes to the child's health, their generalized values about health, attitudes toward doctors, use of medical care, family illness, and their use of medical facilities. Children were interviewed regarding their attitudes toward health and medical facilities and their willingness to report symptoms. The data suggest a small, but significant effect on the child of the mother's attitudes toward health. Children's attentiveness to symptoms were related to those of the mother. At the same time, mothers and children who were very inclined to utilize medical services were both more likely to adopt the "sick role."

These children were followed up by Mechanic in 1979; the aim being to investigate the stability of concepts of health over time. Ninety-five percent of the original sample of 350 children were located. Health-related beliefs did not appear very stable over the 16-year-period, and this applied particularly to areas such as comfort experienced by visiting a doctor or communicating about symptoms with others. In contrast, Mechanic concludes:

> ... there appears to be some continuity in stoicism: young children who do not pay attention to pain are more likely to become adults who deny pain, resist release from life responsibilities when ill, do not discuss their symptoms with others, and are willing to take risks involving possible injury. Risk taking of all the other variables we studied, seems to be most likely to have some stability, but even here the relationship over time is relatively weak. (1979, p. 1144)

In addition to the questions about health-related beliefs, Mechanic (1979) also asked about 10 health-related behaviors in the later study. These included seat-belt use, smoking, risk taking, exercise, enjoyment of physical activity, release (whether the respondent continues with usual activities even when ill), preventive medical care, drinking behavior, physical health, and personal control over illness. Mechanic reports only a low correlation among these behaviors. It is unfortunate that no attempt is made to relate the children's health attitudes on first testing with their health behaviors as adults.

Conclusions

Explanations of the reasons for illness and rationale for medical treatment tend to be dependent on at least some knowledge about the body and how it works as well as basic ideas about disease processes. For this reason alone, the studies reviewed in this section have important practical implications. It is apparent that any adult concerned with explaining illness to a child should not assume a very sophisticated level of knowledge. Further, the child's assumptions about how the body works, or what causes illness, are sometimes potentially erroneous. As such, the child's assumptions can constitute a barrier to understanding. The young child's rigid belief, for example, that all illnesses are caused by being too close to others with illness is likely to make explanations of noncontagious illness especially difficult. In their own study, Kister and Patterson (1980) pointed to the tendency shown by young children to overgeneralize such principles regardless of the etiology of specific diseases.

In this chapter we have reviewed the evidence that children's concepts of their bodies and the causes of illness develop in a predictable fashion, parallel to the acquisition of more physical concepts such as space and time. The approach may be criticized for the almost exclusive dependence on cognitive processes, with little attempt to allow for social or cultural influences. Such criticisms aside, several authors have argued that the schema is sufficiently robust that practical recommendations for communicating with sick children are justified. Bibace and Walsh (1981) for example have gone so far as to suggest that explanations of disease should not be in terms of physiological processes at least until the child reaches the stage of formal operations (i.e., 11 years of age or more). Prior to this they suggest that explanations should focus on more concrete, visible aspects of disease management, such as explanations of medical equipment or differentiation of the role of various medical personnel.

This same developmental schema has been applied by Johnson and co-workers (Harkavy et al., 1983; Johnson et al., 1982) as a guide for offering age-appropriate explanations of diabetes to pediatric patients. This work is considered in more detail in Chapter 6. Such detailed explanations of other diseases have been less, if at all, developed. Yet it is hoped that it is clear that this kind of work has potential practical implications. Developmental studies are limited only by criticisms that could be made of the basic research methods. There are still many questions to be asked about the cognitive processes underlying the child's acquisition of concepts of the body, health, and illness. Research so far has almost all been based on small samples of children. Children's concepts of their bodies have been investigated almost exclusively by asking them to draw their insides, and concepts of illness have been studied almost exclusively by semistructured interviews about the causes of illness. Alternative methods may yield different and more complex views on how these concepts develop. In addition, little attention has been paid to variables that might influence the course of development. Of obvious importance in this respect are social and cultural variables, as well as the child's experience with illness.

Nevertheless, the work reviewed in this chapter is the cornerstone for all that follows. In the remainder of this book, the problems encountered by children in their experiences of hospitals, medical personnel, and procedures, as well as in their attempts to understand specific illnesses and their treatment will be discussed. Our thesis is that, in a wide range of situations, it is difficult to decide what information to give to a sick child, and how to give it. In order that such decisions are not entirely of a trial-and-error kind, it is essential to pursue further research concerned with the normal development of children's concepts of health, illness, and their bodies.

3

Children in the Hospital

Historical Perspectives

Admission to the hospital is a potentially traumatic event for adults and children alike. Hospital buildings are often large and intimidating; patients do not know their way around the maze of corridors and departments. Children are expected to sleep in high cots. Different procedures regarding eating and sleeping habits are expected, and children are likely to be unsure about the behavior to be adopted. In addition, a host of personnel are likely to interact with the child, each performing their own new, often painful, procedure. When we talk about hospital admission affecting a child, we are considering all of these variables together. It is rarely, if ever, possible to separate these variables. Rachman and Phillips (1975) have suggested that it is impossible to distinguish "between the distress caused by admission into hospital and that caused by the illness itself; between the effects of the illness and the medical procedures such as injections, drips, operations and the rest; or between the effects of admission to a *hospital* from the distress which might be caused by a separation from the child's parents" (p. 171). Yet such distinctions "are valuable for heuristic, research, and policy purposes" (Lavigne & Burns, 1981, p. 287).

Despite these difficulties, we should not dismiss research into the psychological effects of hospital admission as trivial. The numbers of children involved are high. Davie, Butler, and Goldstein (1972) found that by 7 years of age, 45% of British children had been hospitalized at least once. More recent statistics (Butler, 1980; Department of Health and Social Security, 1979) found that in a 5-year period, 25.5% of 5-year-olds had been hospitalized at least once.

Before 1952, little attention was paid to identifying any problems for hospitalized children. However, in 1952, Bowlby became concerned with psychological consequences for children of separation experiences. Although the impetus for this work had been on separations during war time, Bowlby chose to study, in addition, separations associated with hospitalization. At the same time Robertson (1952) produced the now classic film called *A Two-Year-Old goes to Hospital*. The film showed the experiences of a little girl throughout her 8-day admission for a hernia operation. The film poignantly captures the child's emotional responses to the experience, moving through the same three stages later described by Bowlby as typical of a child experiencing a break in attachments: protest, despair, and detachment. Gellert (1958) summarized her own observations on hospitalized children as follows:

> The stress of hospitalization for children is manifested in a number of ways. Children cry, whine or scream; they cling tenaciously to their parents; they eat or sleep poorly; they struggle against treatment and resist taking medications; they are tense and fearful; they become silent, sad and withdrawn. They may show an increase in regressive or compulsive behavior, they may become disruptive of their environment, or even themselves.' (p. 171)

That the trauma of such a hospitalization can be reduced by allowing the child's mother to stay throughout the period was emphasized in a later film, *Going to Hospital with Mother* (Robertson, 1958a).

As a result of the growing concern with the experience of hospitalization on a young child, the National Association for the Welfare of Children in Hospitals (NAWCH) was founded in England in 1961. In addition, the British government set up a commission to study the hospitalized child's needs (Platt Committee, 1959). Major changes in pediatric care were recommended by this committee, including the following:

1. Unrestricted visiting by parents to sick children should be encouraged.
2. Mother-and-child units should be established.
3. Children should only be admitted when there is absolutely no alternative.

Four years later, the Nuffield Foundation (1963) financed a study on how children's hospitals could be physically modified so that parents could stay with their children.

Despite the amount of concern that has been shown in Britain for the needs of the hospitalized child and a parallel growth in concern in the United States (Shore & Goldston, 1978), there is still room for considerable improvements in pediatric care. In the most recent survey in England, Thornes (1983) surveyed all acute care wards in the country caring for children under 12 years of age. It was found that 28% of wards in which children were nursed were for adults rather than specifically for children. Despite the recommendations of the Platt (1959) committee that parents should be allowed unrestricted visits to their children, only 49% of wards caring for children had adopted this policy. Eighty-nine percent of wards were still able, however, to provide overnight accommodation for parents. Thornes (1983) concluded that much improvement in the care of hospitalized children had taken place since the Platt Report but considerable improvement could still take place.

The research literature points to hospitalization resulting in behavioral and emotional upset at least for some groups of children. Furthermore, the characteristics of children most at risk following hospital experience have been documented several times. Stacey, Dearden, Pill, and Robinson, (1970) identified vulnerable children as follows:

1. They tended to be only or youngest children from extended families.
2. They tended to respond unfavorably to tests of communicativeness, responsiveness, and aggression.
3. They tended to have mothers who were either especially anxious or bland about hospitals.
4. They responded badly to strange adults or situations.
5. They rarely visited the homes of others.
6. They had recently experienced a traumatic separation, such as starting school or the arrival of a new baby.

The age of the child has consistently been shown to predict reaction to hospitalization. Prugh, Staub, Sands, Kirschbaum, and Lenihan (1953) noted that children under 4 years old showed more persistent signs of emotional disturbance than older children. Schaffer and Callender (1959) reported that babies under 7 months of age did not tend to be adversely affected by hospitalization, presumably because a nurse could substitute the mother's role in these young infants. Studies by Vernon and Schulman (1964) and Vernon, Schulman, and Foley (1966) confirmed the finding that children between 6 months and 4 years of age were more vulnerable following hospitalization than either very young babies or school-aged children. Vernon, Schulman, and Foley (1966) asked mothers of 387 children to complete a Posthospital Behavior Questionnaire. Responses were subject to a factor analysis yielding six dimensions of disturbance: (1) general anxiety and regression, (2) separation anxiety, (3) anxiety about sleep, (4) eating disturbance, (5) aggression toward authority, and (6) apathy–withdrawal. Children aged between 6 months and 4 years scored highest on all six dimensions and especially on the dimension of maternal separation.

Two more recent and large-scale studies broadly confirm these earlier findings. Douglas (1975) investigated a random one-in-four sample of children born in the 1st week of March 1946. Douglas found "strange and unexpected evidence that one admission to hospital of more than a week's duration or repeated admissions before the age of five years (in particular between 6 months and 4 years) are associated with an increased risk of behaviour disturbance and poor reading in adolescence" (p. 476). Douglas further reported that children most vulnerable to hospital admission were those with very dependent relationships with their mothers or those under stress at home at the time of being admitted.

Quinton and Rutter (1976) took advantage of data collected earlier (Rutter 1967; Rutter, Quinton, Rowlands, Yule, and Berger, 1975) to confirm the findings of Douglas (1975). In these studies, all 10-year-old children ($N = 1279$) resident on the Isle of Wight were screened using a teacher's questionnaire designed to identify children with emotional or behavioral problems at school. A similar screening was undertaken 1 year later in one Inner London Borough. Data from these two sources were combined, and 451 children were selected for intensive study. Information about hospital admissions were obtained for 399 of these. Quinton and Rutter found that single hospital admissions of less than 1 week were not associated with later emotional or behavioral disturbance. Repeated hospital admissions, however, did adversely affect development, especially among children from disadvantaged homes. The data did not allow for an analysis in terms of age differences in vulnerability.

In summary, the research literature is fairly consistent in finding some adverse effects on later emotional development for children undergoing hospitalization. The probability of behavior disturbance occurring increases with the number of hospitalizations and for children from disadvantaged backgrounds. Children aged between 6 months and 4 years are more vulnerable than babies or school-aged children. There are few exceptions to these conclusions. Siegel (1974), for example, compared children with a history of hospital admission with their siblings, and found no behavioral differences between them, while Starr (1978) found that hospitalizations did not effect the behavior of preschool children with cleft lip or palette, at least according to mothers' completion of the Missouri Children's Behavior Checklist. The procedure of comparing hospitalized children with healthy siblings has been particularly criticized by Sipowicz and Vernon (1965). These authors investigated twins, where one twin was hospitalized and the other not. There were no significant differences in posthospital behavior between the twins, suggesting that the home twins were as affected by the hospitalization as the siblings.

Several suggestions have been made to reduce the potentially traumatic impact of hospital admission on the child. The Platt report (Platt Committee, 1959) recommended that admissions should only be made when "inescapable." Despite this, Douglas (1975) reported that early admissions during the period 1964–1969 were more frequent than experienced by children in 1946. The length of hospitalization appears to have become significantly less over the 12-year-period, but Douglas found that 9% of children experienced long or repeated admissions in the later period, compared with 7% in 1946.

It is essential, then, to organize a child's stay in the hospital in such a way that the risk of emotional disturbance developing is reduced. As originally recommended in the Platt report, it is becoming more standard practice that the child's mother is encouraged to stay with her child or at least visit as often as possible. Two studies have been specifically addressed to the question of how the presence of a mother affects the child's reaction to hospital. Vernon, Foley, and Schulman (1967) randomly assigned 32 children, aged between 2 and 6 years, to "separate" or "accompanied" conditions. Behavioral observations of the children were made before and after anesthetization. In addition, mothers were interviewed about the child's behavior, and completed the Posthospital Behavior Questionnaire. The degree of stress apparent in children accompanied by their mothers was less than experienced by children alone. In a similar way, Brain and Maclay (1968) compared 101 children admitted to the hospital along with their mothers with 96 admitted alone. The accompanied children were rated as more satis- factorily adjusted during their stay compared with the nonaccompanied children. More emotional disturbance was noted in the nonaccom- panied children following discharge. There would therefore appear to be plenty of support for encouraging parents to accompany their child during admission.

Preparation for Hospital Admission

In addition to encouraging mothers to accompany their children, many workers believe that in order to reduce the stressful experience of hospitalization, children should be prepared for admission beforehand. The rationale is that if a child knows what to expect, less stress will develop. Parents themselves seem unable to prepare their children adequately for the experience. Goffman, Buckman, and Schade (1957) asked 100 children what their parents had told them about why they were coming to hospital. Twenty-six percent had been told nothing, 22% had been given vague reasons, and 27% obtained their information from overhearing others. Only 25% had been adequately prepared according to the authors' criteria. Vaughan (1957) and Levy (1959) found that in many instances parental explanations were so incomplete and far from the truth that the child was subject to even greater stress. The onus is clearly on hospital personnel to provide children with adequate explanations about the reasons for their admissions and the procedures to be experienced.

Most researchers have adopted one of four main types of preparation. Perhaps the simplest involves distributing leaflets informing patients about the hospital generally, or the procedures to be experienced in detail. A second involves home visits by hospital personnel prior to admission, and a third method involves informing the child about procedures (usually surgery) by using video films. Fourthly, and occasionally, play therapy has been used to inform the child.

Play Therapy

Much of a child's anxiety is believed to be reflected in symbolic play (cf., Erikson, 1940; Piaget, 1962). Cassell and Paul (1967) therefore hypothesized that the stress of surgical procedures could be reduced by allowing the child to learn about them during play activities. Twenty children aged between 3 and 11 years and undergoing hospitalization for cardiac catheterization were studied. The children were given two separate 30-minute sessions of puppet therapy. Puppets were made to represent the doctor, nurse, girl, boy, father, and mother. Miniature equipment was used, and the procedures acted out with the puppets. Children's reactions to the procedures themselves were assessed using parental questionnaires, ward observations, and observations during cardiac catheterization. Comparisons were made with 20 children undergoing the same procedures but experiencing routine hospital care.

Children given puppet therapy showed less emotional disturbance during the catheterization procedure, and expressed more willingness to return to the hospital than children given no preparation. However, there were no differences between the groups in emotional disturbances during their hospital stay, or in posthospital behavior. The therapy therefore appears very specific in its value to the children. Nevertheless, it was successful in reducing the stress of the catheterization procedures.

Further support for the value of play therapy was reported by Schwartz, Albino, and Tedesco (1983). They studied 45 children, aged between 3 and 4 years who were hospitalized for dental surgery under general anesthesia. Subjects were randomly assigned to one of three experimental groups. A *control* group received no preoperative preparation. A second group received *unrelated* play therapy, involving a preoperative play session unrelated to surgery. A third group received *related play therapy*. This involved play about hospital and surgical procedures. The child's subsequent behavior was assessed at seven stress points: admission, nurse's examination, pediatric medical examination, blood test, preoperative injection, transfer to surgery, and induction. The related play group showed the least upset behavior, and the control group showed the most. These results were not significant for all of the seven stress points. Related play was superior to unrelated play at only one stress point—induction of anesthesia. This appeared to be the most stressful point for children. The related play group was less upset than the control group at the nurse's examination, preoperative injection, transfer to surgery, and induction. These results are therefore suggestive of the value of play therapy in children undergoing anesthesia. Although there were fewer differences between children in the related and unrelated play groups, such differences as there were occurred at the most severe stress point. Given the potential value of this approach, it is disappointing that so little related work has focused on this aproach. Other work has focused more on the value of video films and home nursing visits.

Video Films

Vernon (1973) used video films to prepare children for anesthesia induction. Half the children were shown a video in which child actors responded calmly to anesthesia. A control group saw no film. The experimental group was rated as showing less fear on induction than the control group. At face value, therefore, this study appears to suggest that by showing children what to expect, fear experienced during anesthetization can be reduced. Perhaps because it was one of the first attempts in this area, however, there were some substantial problems in the research design. It would have been desirable to include a control group who saw a film unconnected with the hospital; perhaps it was simply viewing a film that relaxed the children. In addition, it was only apparent that fear was reduced in relation specifically to anesthesia induction, no data were given to suggest that the children in the experimental condition behaved differently from the control children in other aspects of their hospitalization or on return home.

Vernon and Bailey (1974) attempted to extend these findings, and studied 38 children aged between 4 and 9 years. All children were undergoing minor elective surgery. The preparation film showed "four children responding calmly to mock anesthesia induction" (p. 69). The film was shown 45 minutes before the children underwent anesthesia. Children viewed the film without their parents, but in the presence of the investigator, who commented on the procedures throughout. Children in the control condition waited with their parents and had no contact with the anesthetist or investigator. The mood of the children was rated during the film and on anesthesia induction using the Global Mood Scale. Judgments of the children's behavior were also made by the anesthesiologists. Vernon and Bailey concluded that the prepared children were less upset than unprepared children, both while waiting to enter the operating room and while being prepared for induction. Complicating these conclusions, however, were three anomolies; children in the prepared group were slightly older than those in the unprepared group (6.0 and 5.6 years respectively), more had had previous experience of anesthesia (4 and 2), and there were some differences between the groups in type of anesthesia used. As in the previous study, differences between the groups were only reflected in mood ratings in the period immediately surrounding the induction period, and did not continue for the whole of the child's stay. Although the film was related to differences in children's mood, there were no differences in behavior between the groups according to anesthetist's ratings. The video can therefore only be said to have met with partial success.

Some better-controlled studies were reported by Melamed and colleagues. Melamed and Siegel (1975) investigated 60 children aged between 4 and 12 years. Half the children saw a preparatory film and half a nonpreparatory control film. The group viewing the preparatory film had lower anxiety scores on a variety of measures, and fewer posthospital (1 month after discharge) behavior problems. Melamed, Meyer, Gee, and Soule (1976) were particularly interested in *when* preparation was most likely to be beneficial to children. The authors suggested that older children should benefit from a longer time interval between preparation and surgery, while younger children were more likely to benefit from a shorter separation. (Similar data had previously been reported by Dimock, 1960; Heller, 1967; and Mellish, 1969; Robertson, 1958b). Melamed et al. investigated 48 children aged between 4 and 12 years who were hospitalized for 2–4 days for minor surgery. The children viewed a preparatory film either 1 day prior to admission or 6–9 days prior to admission. Within these groups, half the children also received additional preparation and instruction from nursing staff, and the remainder received standard care.

The results broadly replicated the earlier findings of Melamed and Siegel (1975); children viewing the preparatory film had less self-reported medical concerns and were less anxious according to independent observer's ratings. In addition, these children showed significantly fewer behavior problems on discharge. However, it was not clear that *when* the children viewed the film was predictive of their behavior. There was however, some tendency for older children who viewed the film before admission to show fewer posthospital discharge problems than those who viewed the film immediately prior to surgery. There is clearly an overall beneficial effect of preparing children for hospital using video films. For the future, greater attention needs to be paid to variables such as the optimal time for viewing the film, and how best to modify the content of films for suitability to different age-groups and reasons for admission.

Video Films Combined With Home Visits

Certainly Ferguson (1979) found that preadmission home contact with a nurse was at least as beneficial as showing children video films. Eighty-two children were involved, aged between 3 and 7 years. Again they were hospitalized for 2 days for elective tonsillectomies. In the preadmission group, children were visited 5–7 days prior to admission and given general information about the hospital and how the child might be expected to feel. Mothers were also given a hospital pamphlet. On admission the child and mother were met by the same nurse. Children in the "film" group had no previous contact with hospital personnel or information prior to admission. They were admitted routinely into the hospital (a procedure that lasted 1 hour compared with 5 minutes for the preadmission group). These children were shown a preparatory film called *Yolande and David Have Their Tonsils Out*, while a nonrelated film was shown to the preadmission group.

Ferguson (1979) found age differences in children's responsiveness to the two preparatory techniques. The authors concluded that "the incidence of undesirable post-hospital behavior is most effectively diminished in the younger group by the peer modeling film, while the 6–7 year old group responded as positively to the pre-admission visit" (p. 662). The authors felt that preparation in a visual form (the film) was better for younger children than material in a verbal form (the nurse's home visit). (However, the visual material was presented immediately before surgery and may therefore have had a greater impact for this reason.) Ferguson concluded that either method of preparation is better than standard hospital procedure, but perhaps surprisingly, children who received both methods of preparation did not show further decreases in anxiety or improved posthospital behavior over those just receiving one method of preparation.

A study by Wolfer and Visintainer (1979) sheds some further light on the comparison of effectiveness of different research procedures. In this study 163 children aged between 3 and 12 years, again hospitalized for tonsillectomies, were included. Children were assigned to one of five conditions:

1. Preparatory material at home and routine nursing care in the hospital
2. Stress point preparation in the hospital
3. Home preparatory material plus stress point preparation in the hospital
4. Home preparation plus consistent supportive care from a single nurse in the hospital
5. Routine nursing care

In general the younger patients were more upset and less cooperative than older patients, regardless of the type of preparation. Home preparation did not lead to benefits for mother or child over no preparation, unless it was accompanied by supportive nursing intervention after admission.

Effectiveness of Attempts to Prepare Children for Hospital Admissions

There are three major points to be made in connection with these attempts to prepare children for hospital. The first is that, despite the fact that children aged between 6 months and 4 years are most vulnerable to hospital admission, preparation has mostly been aimed at the 4- to 12-year-old group, with occasional attempts to include 3-year-olds. I suspect that this reflects a bias on the part of researchers rather than an inability on the part of younger children to be prepared at all. Two- to four-year-olds may not be highly receptive to video films, but may well respond to preparation through play. Play therapy may just be a little more difficult and time-consuming to set up.

The second point again centers on the fact that what preparation there is has been directed at the least vulnerable groups of children. Almost without exception, preparation has been aimed at children undergoing short-stay hospitalizations and minor surgery. Yet it is children undergoing long or repeated admissions who are most at risk in terms of subsequent development (cf., Douglas, 1975; Quinton & Rutter, 1976). There remains a desperate need to devise techniques of information-giving that are suitable for children with chronic medical conditions. There are significant numbers of children being treated for conditions such as kidney disease, leukemia, accidents, and burns, who are required to have extended contact with hospitals and medical treatments. The urgent need to devise techniques suitable for preparing children suffering these kinds of conditions has been emphasized by McCue (1980) and Wisely, Masur, and Morgan (1983). These authors were working with patients with leukemia and patients with severe burn injuries, respectively. A recent study by Jay, Ozolins, Elliot, and Caldwell (1983) has demonstrated that it is feasible to prepare leukemia patients for treatment (see Chapter 8). The natural progression for researchers concerned with preparing children for hospitalization must involve greater attention to the needs of the chronically sick and long-stay pediatric patient.

Thirdly, evaluations of techniques to prepare children for hospital have generally been limited to brief (2–4 weeks) posthospital discharge (cf., Melamed & Siegel, 1975; Vernon & Bailey, 1974).

In an attempt to evaluate the effectiveness of preparatory techniques in the long-term, Peterson and Shigetomi (1983) conducted telephone interviews with 40 mothers whose children had been hospitalized 1 year earlier for elective tonsillectomies. All children had received psychological preparation for surgery. Puppet shows, filmed modeling procedures, and training in coping techniques had all been used.

One year after surgery, 67% of mothers interviewed reported that their child still spoke about the hospital admission. Surprising, perhaps, was the finding that while 62% of children spontaneously recalled "positive" aspects of the experience, (e.g., ice cream, electric hospital beds, and color television) only 22% recalled the more negative aspects involving preoperative injections and postoperative pain. Only one mother reported the occurrence of negative behavior changes following discharge.

Peterson and Shigetomi (1983) interpret their data as evidence for the value of preparatory techniques in reducing the incidence of post-hospital anxiety and behavior disturbance. Such a conclusion would only be valid if a control group of children were included who had not received any preparation. The relatively positive effects of hospital admission found in this study may therefore be due to enlightened nursing staff and general attitudes of hospital personnel, rather than preparation per se. Nevertheless, the study does indicate that brief hospitalizations need not be permanently damaging for many children. Indeed, the experience can be regarded in a more positive light than traditionally believed.

Even taking into account these limitations in experimental procedures, it is apparent that attempts to prepare children for hospital admission have met with only partial success. Attempts to prepare the child's parents appear more promising.

Parent Education

Most clinicians recognize, at an intuitive level, differences between parents in their abilities to help their child cope with hospital-related anxieties. Schuster (1951) formalized these ideas and identified three groups of parents, those who instinctively know how to deal with their children's needs because of their own experiences, those who don't know but profit from written or verbal instructions, and those who, because of their own emotional inadequacies, are not able to cope effectively. Schuster suggests that pediatricians need to recognize these differences in their dealings with parents.

In several studies, attempts to prepare mothers for their children's hospital stay appear to have led to improvements in the children's emotional and behavioral responses to hospitalization. Mahaffy (1965) studied 43 children aged between 2 and 10 years and their mothers. Children were assigned to a control group, who received standard admission procedures, or an experimental group, who were helped through admission by a nurse, trained to establish a warm relationship with the mother. There were no differences between the groups on admission. However, during their hospital stay, children in the experimental group showed significantly lower temperatures, blood pressure, and pulse rates. Seven days after discharge mothers were asked to complete a questionnaire covering items such as disturbed sleep, crying, clinging, need to call the doctor, and so on. Children in the experimental group appeared to have made a far better and more rapid recovery on all dimensions.

Similar conclusions were reached by Skipper and Leonard (1968). Half their sample of 80 patients was assigned to a control condition and experienced routine care. The other half was admitted to hospital by a specially trained nurse, who was attentive to the mother's emotional needs. Mothers in the experimental group reported less stress themselves, and this was reflected in improved behavior of their children over those in the control group. Wolfer and Visintainer (1979) also reported the effectiveness of being attentive to parents' emotional needs in reducing the stress experienced by children. In dealing with young children, there is therefore beginning to be evidence that time spent preparing the parents is time well spent. Such a view is endorsed in England by the NAWCH, who suggest that preparation for hospitalization should be directed at the parents rather than the child. However, most researchers do agree that any intervention is better than standard hospital care. Despite this, hospitals vary greatly in the extent to which they use preparation and in the type of technique. Two American surveys have been directed at this question. Peterson and Ridley-Johnson (1980) reported that 70% of nonchronic care pediatric hospitals offered some kind of preparation to parent and child. They noted that 55% distributed coloring or story books, 48% employed play therapy, 37% showed films, 21% held puppet shows, 16% used relaxation training or deep-breathing lessons, and 27% employed procedures such as preadmission tours or acquaintance with medical equipment. It is disheartening to note, however, that even where hospitals offer preparation, many children and parents do not take advantage of it. The survey showed that, on average only 42% of children being admitted actually received some preparation. Parents should begin their teaching about hospitals to children early, so that they are prepared if admission is made. This view may be the best in theory but much education needs to be directed at parents to ensure that they do their part.

A second, and larger survey by Azarnoff and Woody (1981) reported that only 33% of hospitals provided preparation for children. This survey did, however, include both pediatric hospitals and acute care general hospitals. Many of the latter felt that the small number of pediatric patients involved did not warrant the setting-up of preparatory programs. Among those hospitals offering preparation, the most popular techniques prior to admission involved tours and group discussions. Home visits and story books were the least preferred methods. During hospitalization, information was most often given by "learning as events occur" or conversation, with only a small percentage using films. No data were reported as to the numbers of children actually receiving any preparation.

Children's Perceptions of Hospitals

In an earlier review of this literature, Goslin (1978) pointed out the need to integrate findings into a theoretical framework. He argued that preparatory techniques employed were based on one of two theoretical positions. The first centers on the role of cognitive preparation for adequate coping (Janis, 1958). It is assumed that the anxiety surrounding hospitalization can be reduced by creating a degree of stress or "anticipatory worry" beforehand. In this way the individual's defenses are aggravated, and this lessens the impact of the trauma itself. In his own empirical work, Janis concluded that some "work of worrying" was necessary in order for an individual to prepare for a stressful experience.

Although Goslin (1978) was skeptical about the relevance of this theory as applied to children, a study by Burstein and Meichenbaum (1979) suggests that school-aged children, even if not preschoolers, might respond to stress in such a way. Twenty children undergoing minor surgery were studied. Defensiveness (Wallach & Kogan, 1965) and anxiety (Gilmore, 1965) were assessed, both before and 1 week after surgery. In addition, the authors conducted a 7-month follow-up of the children. Dependent measures were the children's relative preference for toys that were or were not relevant to surgery and hospitalization.

Burstein and Meichenbaum (1979) identified two groups of children, differing in the extent to which they engaged in the "work of worrying." The first group had low defensive scores before admission, actively played with stress-related toys, and reported minimal stress and anxiety on discharge. The second group was highly defensive, avoided playing with stress-related toys, and appeared most anxious following surgery. Of interest is the fact that children in the first group recalled significantly more parental statements preparing them for hospital than children in the second group. (This was in spite of the fact that there were no differences between the two groups of parents in the extent to which they reported trying to prepare their children.)

For some children at least, there appear to be parallels with adult coping strategies as described by Janis (1958). Nevertheless, some authors have questioned this type of approach with children, arguing that some children may be more disturbed by attempts at preparation than by the medical procedures themselves (Becker, 1972).

The bulk of the literature concerned with preparing children for hospitalization appears to be based on social learning theory (Bandura & Walters, 1963). In essence, young children exposed to a model showing a behavior new to their repertoire will imitate that behavior. By showing children films of others responding calmly to anesthesia or surgery, the hope is that they will respond in a similar manner. The studies by Ferguson (1979) and Wolfer and Visintainer (1979), for example, represent broad support for this theory. Models who are at first fearful, but overcome this fear and cope effectively, are more successful than models who show no initial anxiety.

Hospital admission is a potential crisis for children. Caplan (1961) has argued that a child may experience such a crisis in one of three ways. Optimally, the individual may learn a new coping strategy, thereby expanding the range of available behaviors and fostering new development. The least desirable outcome is the development of maladaptive coping mechanisms that do not foster growth. A third outcome is that the individual emerges from the crisis unchanged, in which case the child avoids both the potential danger of the situation and also the potential for growth.

A critical determinant of which of the three strategies will emerge appears to be the individual's cognitive interpretation of the event (Hill, 1965). In this way the mother's definition and interpretation of the hospital experience can therefore be seen to be critical in moulding the child's attitudes, a result borne out in empirical studies.

If Goslin's (1978) call for a theoretical approach to preparing children for hospitalization is to be answered, it must be acknowledged that what children need and want to know is dependent on their developmental level. Any approach that does not recognize developmental changes in such needs is doomed to failure. In preparing video films, researchers have tended to decide on the information they feel the child needs and have made one film directed at all age-groups. In fact, we know little about what children themselves think about hospitals or medical procedures, or what aspects they find most distressing. What little research there is suggests that what worries children most may not necessarily be the same as what would worry adults. Perhaps a study by Millstein et al. (1981) is relevant here. In discussing concepts of illness among adolescents, Millstein et al. reported that what was most worrying was the reaction of friends and restrictions of social activities, rather than any pain or fear of hospital procedures.

It is apparent that some very basic research questions need to be answered before effective means of preparing children for hospitalization can occur. If we begin by identifying developmental changes in children's concepts of hospitals and medical procedures, we will be in a far better position to design effective intervention.

In a preliminary study aimed at this question, Eiser and Patterson (1984) interviewed healthy children in schools about their knowledge of what happened in hospitals. Three groups of children were studied; aged 5–6 years, 7–8 years, and 9–10 years. The children were first asked "what would you tell a little boy or girl about what happens in the hospital?" The responses could be coded into one of three categories:

1. *Physical,* involving descriptions of hospital wards and medical procedures
2. *Social,* involving the role of medical staff, presence of other children and visitors
3. *Negative,* involving boredom, loneliness and the possibility of pain or death

While the younger children were as likely to give responses in either the physical or social categories, older children were much more likely to give responses in the social categories. This would parallel the findings of Millstein et al. (1981). These data are summarized in Table 3-1.

A second question concerned what children expected to do all day in hospital. Responses included:

1. *Social,* such as play with other children and interactions with medical staff
2. Stay in bed
3. Read or watch television
4. Boredom
5. Go to the hospital school

For the most part, children expected to stay in bed (see Table 3-2). The two older groups were more likely than the younger group to expect also to play with other children, read, or watch television. They were also more likely to be prepared to be bored. Only two of the children knew of the possibility of going to school.

Thirdly, children were asked how long they expected to stay in the hospital. As shown in Table 3-3, younger children believed that hospital stays were much longer than did the older children. There were also differences in when children believed hospital admission was necessary. Younger children tended to believe that hospital admission occurred for vague, undefined illnesses, while older children were more likely to mention specific diseases. Accidents and broken bones were mentioned by many children.

Fourthly, children were asked what they thought would be the worst thing about being in the hospital. At all ages, a significant number of

Table 3-1. What Would You Tell a Little Boy or Girl About What Happens in the Hospital?

Response	5- to 6-year olds ($n = 21$)	7- to 8-year olds ($n = 24$)	9- to 10-year-olds ($n = 24$)
Physical	17	6	6
Social	21	30	37
Negative	7	5	3

Note. From "Children's perceptions of hospital: A preliminary study" by C. Eiser and D. Patterson, 1984, *International Journal of Nursing Studies, 21.* Reprinted by permission of Pergamon Press, Inc.

children thought that the worst thing would be associated with the pain of the illness or its treatment. However, with increasing age, children were more likely to mention that they would miss friends or the family, be bored, or afraid.

From these data Eiser and Patterson (1984) concluded that children, especially 5- to 6-year-olds, were very ill-informed about what to expect in hospitals. At the same time, children of slightly older ages were as much concerned about social aspects of hospitalization, such as missing school, friends, or parents, as about details of the physical illness and treatment. In conjunction with other data concerned with children's knowledge of health and illness (see Chapter 2), it is apparent that any preparation for hospital admission needs to take account of these social needs of children, in addition to informing them about mechanical details of the treatment. Attempts to prepare children in this way are lacking.

Table 3-2. What Does a Child in the Hospital Have to Do All Day?

Response	5- to 6-year-olds	7- to 8-year-olds	9- to 10-year-olds
Social	4	11	15
In bed	16	20	23
Read/watch TV	10	7	8
Bored	0	4	1

Note. From "Children's perceptions of hospital: A preliminary study" by C. Eiser and D. Patterson, 1984, *International Journal of Nursing Studies, 21.* Reprinted by permission of Pergamon Press, Inc.

Table 3-3. Children's Estimates of Length of Hospital Stay

Length of Stay	5- to 6-year-olds	7- to 8-year-olds	9- to 10-year-olds
Long periods (up to 4 weeks)	8	18	12
Long periods (between 1 and 1000 years)	8	0	2
Depends on illness	0	4	5

Note. From "Children's perceptions of hospital: A preliminary study" by C. Eiser and D. Patterson, 1984, *International Journal of Nursing Studies, 21.* Reprinted by permission of Pergamon Press, Inc.

Children's Ideas About Medical Procedures

An integral part of being hospitalized involves undergoing certain diagnostic procedures that check on the patient's condition and subsequently undergoing treatment to cure the illness. The child is likely to be examined by a doctor and have regular checks made of pulse rate and temperature. Treatments may be by medication, surgery, physiotherapy, diet, or any combination of these and others. While adults may think to offer the child an explanation of the more complex or traumatic procedures (such as surgery), they are less likely to realize that even the more simple procedures need explanations for the young child. Steward and Steward (1981), for example, cite the case of the child who believed that the repeated process of taking his pulse was essential in making him well. Those involved with pediatric leukemia patients will realize that the children often express more anxiety about the relatively simple finger pricks than the more traumatic procedures. Where a child is not offered an explanation for the reasons for a procedure, it is hardly surprising that erroneous beliefs develop. At the same time, it is apparent that explanations of medical procedures to the young child are particularly difficult. It is unfortunately true that pain and discomfort are likely to increase immediately after treatment. For this reason, it is difficult to convey to the young child that such discomfort is desirable for long-term benefit. Small wonder that early reports concluded that children perceived medical treatment as punishment for wrongdoing (Bergmann & Freud, 1965; Eissler, Kris, & Solnitt, 1977; Jackson, 1942; Jessner, Blom, & Waldfogel, 1952; Pearson, 1941).

Later work included the variable of age in considering the child's attitudes to treatment. Peters (1978) for example questioned 24 hospitalized children, and reported that 33% regarded treatment as punishment or hostility. Younger children were more likely to view treatment in this way than older children. The children were also asked to tell stories about treatment. Almost half the children focused on surgery as a means of treatment, even though none of the children were hospitalized for surgery. Treatment for these children was most commonly by ingestion or limitation of activity, yet few children mentioned these methods (7% and 11%, respectively).

Lynn, Glaser, and Harrison (1962) used an interview and structured doll-play situation to compare 25 children with rheumatic fever with 25 children attending a general pediatric clinic. The children were aged between 5 and 11 years. Although Lynn et al. report the numbers of children having anxieties about aspects of the treatment (e.g., injections or surgery), they did not attempt to describe how children thought that various treatments led to recovery. The authors suggested that children may have erroneous ideas about the cause of illness and its treatment, and the authors speculate that these ideas may hinder successful intervention. Anecdotal evidence by Brazelton, Holder, and Talbot (1953) and Schechter (1961) suggest that children are more likely to see treatment as punishment and personnel as wanting to hurt their patients, the longer children remain in the hospital.

One of the few systematic studies was reported by Brewster (1982). She interviewed 50 chronically ill children between 5 and 13 years of age. All children had serious or chronic conditions. An interview was designed to elicit "the ways that the child might view the role of medical personnel and the content of medical procedures." Specific details were not given. Brewster identified three age-related stages in children's cognitions. Between 5 and 6 years of age, all the children studied stated that medical procedures were done to punish them for bad behavior. For all children, the beneficial effects of treatment occur after the painful medical procedures, so it is perhaps unreasonable to expect any other response. Particularly for chronically sick children, who undergo many procedures but experience little positive improvement, such responses should be even less surprising.

Between the ages of 7 and 10 years, children do become aware of the true purpose of medical treatment. Although Brewster found that children of this age believed that the purpose of medical treatment was to make them better, they did not credit doctors and nurses with an awareness of the painful aspects of treatment. They believed that doctors could only realize that children were in pain if they cried.

Children over 10 years old were found to be able to infer the purpose of medical treatment and to realize that medical staff were aware of the painful nature of treatment even if the child did not cry. Despite this level of reasoning, some children still believed that doctors could not really know how they felt because personal experience was necessary.

In the study by Beales et al. (1983) reported in the previous chapter, children with chronic rheumatoid arthritis were asked about their beliefs regarding the role of therapy. Children aged between 6 and 11 years could not comprehend that treatments with immediate unpleasant effects could have any beneficial long-term consequences. Thus, they assumed that nice-tasting medicine must be good for you, since its effect was immediate in producing a pleasant experience to counter the pain of the disease. Nasty-tasting medicine was felt to do more harm than good because it added to the immediate distress of the illness. In the same way, many 6- to 11-year-olds saw no point in taking tablets that had no agreeable taste and were often difficult to swallow. Children in this age-range assumed that tablets finished up in their stomachs, and they therefore could see no mechanisms whereby swallowing tablets could alleviate pain in the joints. Neither did these children understand how injections could relieve their pain. Rather, injections were perceived as yet another assault on the body. In contrast, older children appeared more appreciative of the fact that unpleasant treatment might have long-term benefits.

All the work reviewed above has focused on the beliefs about medical treatment given by severely ill children. For the majority of children, their experiences of hospitals is usually limited to brief in- or outpatient visits. The expectations that children bring to these situations are likely to determine their cooperation and be of particular importance in dealing with sudden or traumatic injury. The work by Steward and associates (Steward & Steward, 1981) highlights how children can misperceive the reasons for even the very simple and everyday medical procedures.

Steward and Regalbuto (1975) investigated children's knowledge of two instruments commonly used in medical assessments, a stethoscope and a syringe. The children were encouraged to use the instruments to find out what was wrong with one of the authors, a 1st-year medical student. Two groups of children took part in the study, 6- and 8-year-olds. Most children apparently used the stethoscope first on themselves, putting the earpiece in their ears and listening to their own chests. The 6-year-olds believed the function of the stethoscope to be to determine if the patient were alive or dead. Older children were more likely to acknowledge that the doctor was listening to *how* the heart was beating, rather than whether it was beating at all. None of the children used the syringe to give themselves an injection, but they did give one to the medical student.

Steward and Regalbuto (1975) concluded that children did not perceive all medical procedures as alike. Their behaviors with the syringe were cautious compared with their behavior with the stethoscope. The younger children particularly disliked the use of the syringe, and on the whole they did not understand that the syringe contained medicine. Steward and Regalbuto found that even if the children were persuaded that the syringe contained medicine, they could not see how this could enter the body. As far as they were concerned, only the needle entered. At a cognitive level, Steward and Regalbuto concluded that children understood the rationale for medical procedures according to the limitations that would be predicted from Piagetian developmental theory. (Piaget, 1970)

Conclusions

Work by Bowlby (1952) emphasized that hospitalization was a traumatic experience for the child. Children's reactions could be categorized into three stages: protest, despair, and detachment. Largely as a consequence of Bowlby's work, greater attention was given to the psychological needs of the child in hospital (Platt Committee, 1959). As a result, it has become much more accepted that parents (usually mothers) can accompany their child throughout the experience.

A second change in policy has focused on trying to reduce the anxiety and fear associated with hospitalization by devising techniques to prepare the child. Three methods were identified; play therapy, use of video films, and use of home visits by medical personnel prior to admission. The conclusion of this and previous reviews (cf., Ferguson, 1979) is that any method of preparation is superior to no preparation at all. Much remains to be learned, however, about how variables such as the timing of the intervention and content of the films can be modified to increase success.

It must be noted that interventions have not generally been directed at the groups most in need. Very young children (under 4 years old) have often been ignored, despite the well-established finding that hospitalization is particularly traumatic for this group (Prugh et al., 1953; Vernon & Schulman, 1964). Neither has much attention been given to the needs of the chronically sick child, undergoing repeated admissions and procedures (McCue, 1980). Finally, little attention has been given to the needs of the adolescent, whose vulnerability may well be greater than has generally been believed (Shore & Goldston, 1978).

I began this chapter by stating that it was not possible to distinguish between factors such as parental separation, hospitalization, treatments or illness, and their consequences for the child. In fact, the confusion is between the effects of hospitalization and acute illness; previous literature has paid only lip service to the needs of chronically sick children. The special circumstances of these children are considered more fully in the next chapter.

4

Effects of Chronic Illness on the Child, Family, and Siblings

Chronic illness in a child is a diagnosis that affects the whole family. In this chapter, I review previous research into the effects of chronic illness on the child and the family. Wherever possible, the aim is to emphasize the extent to which knowledge of the disease and perceptions of its limitations determine a family's coping style.

Effects of Chronic Illness on the Child

Variables that determine how a child reacts to a diagnosis of chronic illness have generally been grouped in three broad categories (Lavigne & Burns, 1981; Lipowski, 1970; Pless & Pinkerton, 1975). These include

1. *Disease-related factors*, including the severity and chronicity of the illness, and the restrictions thereby placed on the child's life
2. *Intrapersonal factors*, including the child's personality, intelligence and social background
3. *Environmental factors*, including the attitudes of parents and others to the illness

Results from the three epidemiological surveys described in Chapter 1 (Pless & Douglas, 1971; Pless & Roghmann, 1971; Rutter, Graham, & Yule, 1970) suggest that children with chronic illness are at greater risk of developing emotional, social, and behavior problems than healthy children. The risk is not identical for all chronically sick children, however. In both the studies by Pless and Roghmann (1971) and Rutter, Graham, and Yule (1970), it was reported that children with sensory disorders had higher levels of maladjustment than those with motor or cosmetic disorders. More problems were also found for those with permanent rather than temporary disabilities resulting from illness. Results of this kind indicate that children with chronic illness should not be considered a homogeneous group; some account needs to be taken of the idiosyncratic limitations and difficulties posed by different illnesses. Reviews by Lipowski (1970), Pless and Pinkerton (1975), and Lavigne and Burns (1981) describe some of the disease-related factors thought critical in determining the child's adjustment. While most of these factors make intuitive sense, there is not always much related empirical work.

Disease-Related Factors

Severity

Linde, Rosof, Dunn, and Rabb (1966), working with children with congenital heart disease, and O'Malley, Koocher, Foster, and Slavin (1979), working with survivors of childhood cancer, found no relationship between severity of illness and degree of maladjustment. There are, however, several studies that conclude that the *least* severely afflicted children tend to be more maladjusted than those suffering more severe illnesses and disabilities. This applies, for example, to partially hearing compared with deaf children (Rodda, 1970; Sussman, 1966; Williams, 1970) and to partially sighted compared with blind children (Cowen, Underberg, Verillo, & Benham, 1961). Those more severely affected by juvenile arthritis (McAnarney, Pless, Satterwhite, & Friedman, 1974), thalidomide (McFie & Robertson, 1973), and hemophilia (Bruhn et al., 1971) have been shown to be less maladjusted than children with milder forms of the illness. In attempting to explain these results, Wright (1960) has argued that the more severely affected children recognize their limitations and do not attempt to compete with their normal peers. Less severely affected individuals attempt to function in both the world of the normal child and that of the sick child, and this "imagined status" leads to conflict and reduced effectiveness of functioning. The child's constant failure to achieve in the normal world results in a poor self-image and subsequent inadequate adjustment. An alternative hypothesis has been put forward by Garson, Benson, Ivler, & Patton (1978). They argue that children with less severe handicaps are at greater psychological risk because their parents are perceived to need less support than they in fact do, a hypothesis that should be readily verifiable.

Chronicity

A simple prediction might be that psychological maladjustment increases with the length of time since diagnosis of the disease.

Certainly, number of hospitalizations, amount of missed schooling, and financial stresses may well increase. In practice, no reports of such a simple relationship have been made. Rather, there is some evidence that problems are most likely to occur around the time of diagnosis, perhaps then subsiding and reemerging at times of later crisis or the child's death. Longitudinal studies on the psychological effects of leukemia support this view (Schulman & Kupst, 1980).

Unpredictability of course of the disease

With some diseases the child's condition is likely to be stable and to show little day-to-day fluctuation (e.g., in some orthopedic conditions). In others, there can be considerable variability. MacCarthy (1975) interviewed mothers of children with leukemia. The women reported that they underwent increases in stress and anxiety immediately before hospital appointments. As children with leukemia generally attend hospital for checkups at 3-week intervals, it is clear that the pattern of stress created is likely to be intense, and this probably applies to the child as well as the mother. In other conditions, such as diabetes, epilepsy or hemophilia, there can be considerable unpredictability about the child's condition from day to day. While it might be expected that this lack of predictability could be aversive for the family, there are no comparative studies designed to test the hypothesis.

Demands of the treatment regime

The demands of caring for a sick child can be enormous, and most chronic illnesses involve much home treatment by parents. At best, this can be limited to administering pills each day (as in the case of well-controlled leukemia). Even this relatively simple task, though, can assume disproportionate importance, especially when the child has already undergone much treatment (MacCarthy, 1975). Conditions such as diabetes involve daily monitoring of blood and urine and administering appropriate insulin injections. Craig (1982) has described family's responses to these demands. Burton (1975) studied the effects on family life of having a child with cystic fibrosis and concludes that treatment demands, such as daily physiotherapy, are time-consuming and create hardship. Practical problems in dealing with a child with renal failure are described by Korsch et al. (1973). Most research is consistent in finding that it is especially during adolescence that children resent the demands made by their treatment. During adolescence children are likely to resent their extended dependence on adults. Reports of noncompliance with medical treatment have been made for diabetics (Mattson & Gross, 1966; Mattson, Gross, & Hall, 1971) and cystics (Pinkerton 1974; Tropauer, Franz & Dilgard, 1970).

Other disease-related variables suggested by Lavigne and Burns (1981) include the following:

1. *Visibility*. Where an illness affects physical appearance or movements, there is potentially greater threat to the individual than for "hidden" diseases.
2. *Isolation*. Disorders involving isolation (for the purposes of treatment) or because of sensory impairment (as in blindness) are thought to be more likely to lead to maladjustment.
3. *Pain*. Greater pain would be expected to lead to greater maladjustment.

It seems possible to extend such a list indefinitely, but lack of much convincing empirical support makes it unjustified.

Intrapersonal Factors

Age at onset of disease

There is a general finding in the research literature that the adverse consequences of chronic illness are potentially greater the younger the child on diagnosis. Maddison and Raphael (1971) have suggested that qualitatively different consequences of illness develop depending on the child's age at diagnosis. Where illness occurs in a child under 3 years old, there will be a limitation on the child's opportunity for self-expression, an increase in maternal control, and a resultant increase in passive and helpless behavior. Children developing illness between 4 and 6 years of age are likely to develop extreme guilt and inhibition of initiative. Illness developing between 6 and 11 years of age may result in a sense of inadequacy and insecurity, and illness beginning during adolescence is most likely to interfere with the establishment of role and identity.

In fact, there is little evidence for anything but a simple correlation between poorer outcomes in both behavioral and intellectual terms, the younger the child on diagnosis. Williams (1970) for example found that the younger deaf children were on diagnosis, the poorer their subsequent adjustment. Taylor and Falconer (1968) and Gudmondsson (1966) studied adults with temporal lobe epilepsy and concluded that the rate of psychiatric referral was higher for those experiencing their first seizure during childhood, rather than adulthood. An exception is a study by Shaffer, Chadwick, and Rutter (1975), who did not find any association between age of injury and rate of psychiatric referral among children sustaining head injuries between 6 months and 12 years of age.

Several studies also suggest that intelligence is likely to be more compromised among children developing chronic illness early in life. This has been reported for diabetics by Ack, Miller, and Weil (1961); for epileptics by Dikmen, Mathews, and Harley, (1975); and for children with leukemia by Eiser and Lansdown (1977) and brain tumors by Eiser

(1981). Explanations have centered on the fact that the young child's brain is less developed and is immature compared with the older child's (Dobbing, 1974). It has been suggested that such immaturity renders the child's brain more likely to physical damage by the disease and its complications (Ack et al., 1961) or results from iatrogenic effects of treatment (Eiser & Lansdown, 1977).

Other variables that might determine the child's adjustment to chronic illness have been less well-researched. There is a little evidence to suggest that the more *intelligent* child is more adaptive in dealing with the illness (Vignos et al., 1972). Hardy (1968) reported that, among a group of blind children, those with higher IQ scores had lower measures of anxiety. Other work suggests that good adjustment is associated with higher *social class*, at least among blind children (Cowen et al., 1961). It is possible that socioeconomic factors mask some other variables that actually account for this finding. Whether this may be the education level of the parents, increased financial resources, or some other related variable has not been clarified. That these variables contribute to maladjustment in the child is however, beyond questioning. Seidel, Chadwick, and Rutter (1975) studied children with neuroepileptic conditions. A significant association was found between the presence of psychiatric disorder in the child and the following: marital discord, broken home, crowded living conditions, and maternal (but not paternal) psychiatric disorder. Rutter (1977), in a related report, again concluded that there was an increase in psychiatric disorders for children with physical disabilities and poor psychosocial situations compared with those in better psychosocial circumstances. Pless, Roghmann, and Haggerty (1972) developed a "family functioning" index, based on interview ratings of marital satisfaction, frequency of disagreements, family happiness, parental communication, discussion of problems, and free time spent together. Chronically ill children from poorly functioning families were at greater risk in terms of developing maladjustment problems than children from better functioning families.

Environmental Factors

Surprisingly little empirical work has been conducted on the question of how parent–child interaction is modified when the child suffers a chronic or fatal illness. This is particularly surprising in that there has been considerable interest in the relationship between other "risk" factors in the child and mother–infant interaction. Probably widest interest has focused on family interactions following the birth of a premature baby. Mothers of premature babies are generally characterized as making greater effort to engage the child in social interaction, while at the same time the premature baby shows less response than that of the full-term, healthy infant (Brown & Bakeman, 1979; Field, 1977). Parents of premature babies initially make less body contact with the child (Divitto & Goldberg, 1979; Klaus, Kennel, Plumb, & Zuehlke, 1970; Leifer, Leiderman, Barnett, & Williams, 1972), spend less time face to face (Klaus et al., 1970), smile at the infant less (Leifer et al., 1972), touch less, and talk to them less (Goldberg, 1979). While some reports have not found that differences between mother's interactions with premature and normal babies persist (Goldberg, Brachfeld, & Divitto, 1980), other have shown that qualitative aspects of interaction are significantly affected for some time (Beckwith, Cohen, Kopp, Parmelee, & Marcy, 1976; Beckwith, & Cohen, 1978). Bidder, Crowe, and Gray (1974) reported that mothers of premature babies persisted in describing the children as weak even at 3 years of age. This perception was influenced as much by maternal anxiety at the time of birth as the child's physical status.

Such differences in perception are important because they probably determine parents' behavior toward the child. A study of children misdiagnosed with cardiac disease may serve to illustrate this point. Cayler, Lynn, and Stein (1973) found that 34 healthy children incorrectly diagnosed in this way had depressed developmental test scores. A subgroup of nine children who were wrongly diagnosed and placed on restricted activity had even lower IQ scores. The authors suggest that parents impose restrictions on the child's activities in response to the diagnosis, and this results in lower scores. (Reassessments of the child's progress following parents' realization of the misdiagnosis would seem an appropriate extension of this work.)

Much relevant work has also been conducted into mother–child relationships where the child is deaf. Schlesinger and Meadow (1972) found that mothers of hearing children were more permissive, flexible, nonintrusive, and encouraging or approving than mothers of deaf children. Both Collins (1969) and Goss (1970) reported that mothers of deaf children were more "directing" than normal mothers. Meadow (1975) attributes part of the reason for these differences in behavior to the tendency to place more responsibility for the child's education on the mother of the deaf child compared with a hearing child. Mothers of the deaf are trained to be the child's educator, and the strains accompanying this are added to the everyday burdens of child rearing.

Wedell-Monnig and Lumley (1980) observed the behavior of six normal mother–infant pairs and six pairs in which the child was deaf. The children were aged between 13 and 29 months and visited the laboratories on four occasions over a 2-month period. The deaf children were more passive and less actively involved in interactions than the hearing children. In addition, the mothers of the deaf children tended to be more dominant. The most disturbing finding of the study was that older deaf children and their mothers were less involved with each other than younger deaf children and mothers. For normal hearing pairs, the results were in exactly the opposite direction, i.e., the older children were more involved. Wedell-Monnig and Lumley advance two hypotheses to account for their results. Following Schlesinger and Meadow (1972), they suggest that the mother of a deaf child may flood the child with stimulation in order to compensate for the handicap. This may lead ultimately to the child making no contribution to the interaction, since the mother controls it so completely. The alternative hypothesis, which they favor, is in terms of the learned helplessness theory of Seligman (1975). They suggest that with age, the deaf child's ideas and needs increase in complexity, while communicative ability remains immature. This failure to communicate accurately results in the child feeling helpless and ultimately passive and undemanding in interactions. Similar conclusions have been reached by Henggeler and Cooper (1983).

The central role of parental attitudes and behavior toward a chronically sick child have been noted by Freeman (1968). He suggested that a child is most likely to make a good adjustment to chronic illness where the parents adopt a positive, accepting approach to the child. Other work suggests that the child's adjustment does indeed reflect that of the parents (McFie & Robertson, 1973; Tropauer, Franz, & Dilgard, 1970). The difficulties and dilemmas faced by parents in creating such a "positive" climate should not be trivialized, however. Lavigne and Burns (1981) summarize the dilemma as follows:

> The "accepting" climate cannot be overdone, however. For the child to adjust well to an illness or handicap, it is widely recognized that the parent must still make the necessary demands upon the child for appropriate behavior toward peers and siblings, independence training, and developing the ability to tolerate the frustration that accompanies efforts towards academic achievement. In the healthy environment, there must be a balance between recognizing ("accepting") the child's limitations while maximizing the child's strength and skills whenever possible. (p. 310)

Four deviant patterns of parent–child interaction have been identified as follows:

1. Hostile-rejecting relationships
2. Overindulgence
3. Disruptions in attachment formation
4. Overprotectiveness

The dilemma for parents may be summarized in the following quotation from Goodall (1976) "... we don't mind her being a bit spoilt, but we wouldn't want her ruined" (p. 86).

Once again, the amount of empirical work available to substantiate these essentially clinical observations is negligible. There have been a few attempts to infer qualitative aspects of parent–child interaction from interview studies with parents, and even fewer attempts to observe directly interactions between parents and their sick children. Interview studies include those by Barsch (1968), working with parents of the blind and deaf and those with cerebral palsy and Down's syndrome, and Hewett, Newson, and Newson (1970), working with parents of children with cerebral palsy. Both concluded that, according to parents' reports, the child's condition had not led to significant changes in patterns of interaction. Linde, Rosof, Dunn, and Rabb (1966) reported a correlation between maternal overindulgence and anxiety and adjustment problems in the child. (The design of this study was not such that it was possible to establish if maternal attitudes produced adjustment problems in the child, or whether the child's behavior led to adverse maternal attitudes.)

That the child's physical appearance can determine the parents' attitude to the child is shown in studies of children with short stature. Parents tend to relate as to a much younger child. Gordon, Crouthamel, Post, and Richman (1982) showed that parents of children with short stature had less strict approaches to child rearing than parents of same-aged normal children. These families also showed lower levels of cooperation and communication than among normal families.

One of the first attempts to observe parent–child relationships in this context was by Shere (1957). The children were twins, where one twin suffered from cerebral palsy and the other was normal. Mothers were more directive to the child with cerebral palsy, and consequently this child was less involved in family decisions.

Other workers have stressed the demands made on families by the amount of home treatment involved in the care of the child with cystic fibrosis. This includes antibiotic medication, mist tent therapy, and daily postural drainage treatments (Allan, Townley, & Phelan 1974; McCollum & Gibson, 1970). These demands have been found to create difficult child-rearing dilemmas for parents (Allan et al., 1974; McCollum & Gibson, 1970; Meyerowitz & Kaplan, 1967; Turk, 1964).

Kucia et al. (1979) used home observation of parent–child interaction to investigate the relationship between the quality of this interaction and the child's adjustment to cystic fibrosis. Families were involved in two structured tasks in their home. In the first, the Unrevealed Differences Technique (Ferreira & Winter, 1968), each family member was to fill out a questionnaire about individual likes and dislikes. As a group, the family then completed the same questionnaire. A measure of "openness of communication" was devised, reflecting any difference between what a person said in the family group compared with individual responses.

The second task was a "Simulated Family Activity Game" (Straus & Tallman, 1971). Families were given a motor task and were to work together to discover the rules of the game. The following measures of family interaction were obtained: (1) family success at the game, (2) creativity (the number of different ways of playing the game originated by each person), (3) support (classified as positive or negative).

The results suggested that family creativity was particularly associated with better adjustment in the child. The authors suggest that creativity may be important in the management of chronic disease. In that management requires a complex series of adjustments to balance the needs of the sick child with those of other family members, such creativity may be essential.

Further evidence of the importance of family functioning in the adjustment of the child with cystic fibrosis was reported by Lewis and Khaw (1982). Using paper-and-pencil assessments of family functioning, they concluded that adjustment problems in the children were more related to family functioning than the presence of the disease.

These studies have focused on mother–child interaction in situations where the child suffers a chronic or life-threatening condition. McCormick, Shapiro, and Starfield (1982) suggest that minor illnesses in the child can influence the mother's perceptions of the child and subsequently her expectations regarding development. These authors interviewed a total of 4,989 mothers, including a high number (3,179) who had a child of low birth weight. The relationship of the mother's opinion of the development of the child at 1 year was related to differences in sociodemographic, antenatal, intrapartum, and infant health variables. In addition, the child's gross motor development was assessed at the interview. Among infants considered to be developing at a normal rate, 4.0% were considered to be developing slowly by mothers. Among those who were developing more slowly, 28.6% were considered by their mothers to be developing slowly. For both groups, mothers' opinion was largely influenced by infant health status including factors such as low birth weight, congenital anomalies regardless of severity, hospitalization during the 1st year of life, and high ambulatory care use. McCormick et al. conclude that maternal perceptions of the child's health do not reflect actual health, but rather the incidence of past or present illness. In that such conclusions can be reached by studying infants with relatively minor health problems and essentially normal development, it is clear that more significant effects are likely to occur with more severely ill children. Much more work is needed to understand the processes whereby parental perceptions are distorted following childhood illness. In addition, the link between these perceptions and subsequent behavior and development in the child, which has been speculative in the past, needs empirical verification.

Assessing the Effects of Chronic Illness on the Child

Traditionally, there have been four approaches to assessing the impact of chronic illness on the child (Pless & Pinkerton, 1975). The child's *intellectual* or *academic* status has been considered a good indicator by many. Secondly, the child's *social adjustment* can be assessed. Longer-term sequelae have been measured in terms of an individual's *marital* or *occupational* status.

Intellectual Status

Although some illnesses are known to damage the developing brain, the majority of chronic illnesses in childhood are not thought to cause physiological damage as such. It could therefore be argued that chronically sick children should not differ from healthy children in terms of IQ scores or any other indicators of academic achievement. In practice, however, it is apparent that the life-style of the chronically sick child is not likely to be maximally conducive to academic prowess. The sick child is likely to have a poorer school attendance record (Eiser, 1980b; Taylor & Falconer, 1968). In many cases, school attendance is likely to be interrupted for frequent but brief periods, a situation that is potentially more disruptive than a single extended period of absence (Rutter, 1975). Even when he or she is in school, the chronically ill child may feel sleepy or generally under the weather as a result of drugs used to control the disease. Instances of both parents (Burton, 1975) and teachers (Greene, 1975) changing their expectations about the child's attainments have been noted. Reports have consistently concluded that chronically sick children have IQ scores within the normal range, but that their academic achievements are considerably lower than would be expected from age-related norms. Early work was reviewed by Pless and Pinkerton (1975). In addition, work relating to the intellectual and academic status of children suffering from diabetes, asthma, leukemia, and phenylketonuria will be considered in the relevant chapters.

The use of an IQ score as an indicator of the child's adjustment to chronic illness has been criticized. The main objection centers on the argument that IQ tests are not sufficiently sensitive to detect changes that might be attributable to illness or drug effects (St. James Roberts, 1979). Nonetheless, such measures continue to be used by many researchers.

Social and Personality Measures

Most work has focused on the child's personality (as measured by paper-and-pencil tests, projective measures, or interview) and behavior in school and at home. The most popular personality measures include anxiety (Waechter, 1971), hostility or aggression (Downing, Moed, & Wright, 1961; Green & Levitt, 1962; Lipsett, 1958), and self-concept (Piers & Harris, 1964).

Several measures have been devised to assess the child's behavior in school and home. In England, Rutter (1967) has developed the most widely used scales. The Teacher's Behaviour Questionnaire (Rutter, 1967) consists of 26 statements rated as "certainly applies," "applies somewhat," and "doesn't apply" (scored as 2, 1, and 0, respectively). Items such as "fidgets, bites nails, truants, steals" are included. The scale has been used to study children with phenylketonuria (Stevenson et al., 1979), asthma (Graham, Rutter, Yule, & Pless, 1967), uncomplicated epilepsy (Rutter, Graham, & Yule, 1970), and brain lesions (Seidel et al., 1975). The questionnaire has been criticized for relying exclusively on negative personality traits. Although Weir and Duveen (1981) have developed a related scale, biased toward positive traits, it has been used far less extensively. It must also be remembered that the scale was devised and normalized for 9-year-old English children. In studies where it has been used with sick children, the scale has been applied to children across a range of ages, a procedure that may not be entirely justified. Nevertheless, scales devised by Stott (1966) and Conners (1969) are also in use. Richman and Graham (1971) have also published a scale designed to look at behavior problems among 3-year-olds. Despite its potential use in assessing sick preschoolers, the scale has not yet been used in this way.

Marital Status

Pless and Pinkerton (1975) suggested that a third indicator of adjustment to normal life following a chronic illness was an individual's marital or sexual status. Little work has, however, been published in this area. Such research as there is suggests that marriage rates are lower among those with a history of severe illness or handicapping conditions compared with healthy individuals. This has been reported by Brieland (1967), studying students with orthopedic handicaps; Lambert, Hamilton, and Pellicore, (1969), studying a group of amputees; Katz (1963), studying hemophiliacs; Rainer, Altschuler, and Kallman (1963), studying the deaf; and Lindsay, Ounsted, and Richards (1979), studying a group who had suffered temporal lobe seizures since childhood.

Increasing success in treating childhood cancers has led to the survival of a group who are believed to be cured but did nevertheless experience a very disturbed unnatural childhood during the course of their treatment. In addition, cancer is such an emotive disease that it is very necessary to consider how well rehabilitated such people are. Holmes and Holmes (1975) investigated 124 individuals who had survived at least 10 years following treatment for cancer. Sixty of the sample had married, although eight of these were already divorced. Of 41 individuals who had never married, 36 stated that their reason for not marrying was directly related to the disease or its resulting disability. Among those who had married, 34 had children, but 6 were sterile. One patient actually stated that he did not intend to have children because he believed there might be a risk related to his cancer.

Although there is often no reason why individuals with a chronic illness should not marry, their chances of marriage are determined as much by the attitudes of society as by their own inclinations. The low rates of marriage reported may therefore be considered a function of the public's prejudices. This same objection can be raised against the fourth outcome status described by Pless and Pinkerton (1975), namely, an individual's occupational status.

Occupational Status

Unfortunately, individuals with a history of serious illness or resulting disability are less likely to be in permanent employment and more likely to hold manual rather than professional positions than are comparable groups of healthy individuals. This has been reported by M. Vernon (1969) dealing with the deaf, and by Katz (1963), dealing with hemophiliacs. Some employment is thought inadvisable for individuals with certain illnesses. Diabetics, for example, would not be encouraged to undertake work involving great heights (such as on scaffolding or as crane drivers), dangerous machinery, driving public service vehicles, and flying. In general, the British Armed Forces, police, and fire-brigades only employ diabetics in sedentary positions (Tattersall & Jackson, 1982). Diabetics are generally advised to take jobs in which energy expenditure and mealtimes are predictable. Although this ought to enable the diabetic a reasonable choice in career, there are still objections on the part of employers, particularly in times of recession, when "healthy" individuals can be employed as easily. Employers are concerned about absenteeism, accident-proneness, and complications with insurance and superannuation schemes, which are created by employing a "sick" person. Difficulties encountered by the diabetic in gaining employment have been described by Tattersall and Jackson (1982).

A recent study of young adults suffering since childhood from juvenile arthritis (Miller, Spitz, Simpson, & Williams, 1982) is more optimistic. Of 121 adults traced, 45 were working full-time, 25 were in school full-time, 23 were in school and working, and 14 were married women at home. There were no differences between these patients and their siblings in terms of mean educational level or financial income.

Effects of Chronic Illness on the Family

Chronic illness in a child challenges the family at three levels (Sargent, 1982). First there is the *cognitive* challenge. The family must learn about the cause of the illness, its prognosis, complications, and the routines and reasons for the treatment. The family must revise its expectations for the daily life of the sick child, both for the present and the future, and attempt to match the child's activities with the limitations of the disease and treatment. It is up to the family to assign illness management tasks to the child appropriate for age and developmental status, while maintaining responsibility for many other aspects of monitoring the disease.

The second challenge is *emotional*. For the family, this involves coming to terms with anxieties and uncertainties of the illness including, for many, the fear that the child's condition is likely to deteriorate. For the child, there is a need to accept an increased dependency on others, both on parents and medical personnel. Changes in body appearance or function must be responded to, and limitations of treatment accepted. The child is likely to be approached differently by peers, to be prevented from certain activities, and likely to suffer a deduction in self-esteem as a consequence. For many children there may also be a growing awareness of the self as a source of continuing pain and burden to the rest of the family.

Finally, chronic illness presents a *behavioral* challenge. Treatment regimens and hospital visits must be incorporated into the family's way of life while at the same time preserving other family functions, and enabling the family to carry out other essential tasks. The family must also recognize changes in the sick child's ability to perform some tasks and should help where necessary.

While a considerable amount has been written describing a family's initial reactions to learning that a child has a chronic illness, considerably less attention has been paid to the question of how family dynamics and behaviors change during the course of the illness. Paradoxically, there has also been a substantial interest in the family's reactions to the death of a child and subsequent bereavement.

The process of initial adjustment has been described in terms of progressive stages (Kübler-Ross, 1969). There is an initial phase of *shock*, usually described as a protective mechanism and lasting only a brief time. This is followed by a phase of *denial*. This phase may be more prolonged and serves to protect the individual and family from the implications of the illness. *Anger* may parallel or follow denial. It may be directed at family, professionals, or God and is a response to the unfairness of the situation and the fact that an individual is forced to make changes in life-style through no personal fault. At any stage, *depression* can set in. This may reflect the patient's perception of a hopeless and unrewarding life, or guilt about the cause of the illness or unexpressed anger. In discussing chronic illness within a family, Kessler (1977) subsumes all these phases within the diagnostic period. Of much longer duration is the following *adaptive* phase, in which patient and family learn to accommodate to the illness and function within the limits set by the illness.

Moos and Tsu (1977) argue that adaptation to illness consists of a series of skills acquisitions. The patient is thus seen as very actively involved in the process of adaptation. The first category of skills is based on minimizing or denying the seriousness of the illness. This is followed by a set of skills consisting of seeking relevant information and learning about the illness. A third involves requesting reassurance and emotional support from family, friends, and professionals. The fourth is learning specific illness-related procedures (e.g., insulin injections or urine testing for diabetics, physiotherapy for patients with cystic fibrosis). The fifth involves setting up realistic goals and breaking difficult tasks down into manageable parts. Sixth, patients must consider alternative outcomes and develop strategies for coping with them. Finally, patients must find a new purpose in living and put ambitions and behaviors into perspective.

While chronic illness represents a crisis for the family, many families appear to be able to resolve the crisis to an impressive degree. Steinhauer, Mushin, and Rae-Grant (1974) have listed the following variables that influence the family's response to the illness:

1. The severity of illness, its prognosis, and the effectiveness of available treatment
2. Whether the disease is congenital or acquired
3. The child's age at diagnosis
4. Any preexisting emotional disturbance within the family
5. The effects of the illness (including physical changes such as loss of limbs or disfigurement)
6. Restrictions on family life imposed by the disease and its treatment
7. Whether or not other siblings are affected
8. The occurrence of repeated hospitalization and surgical procedures
9. The financial cost of the illness

Thus, each major illness exerts its own idiosyncratic problems on the family. Hemophilia, for example, is a life-threatening disease, transmitted genetically from mother to son. How the mother copes with this knowledge is central to the family's adjustment. Because of the inherited nature of the disease, it is likely that the mother remembers the sufferings of another male relative in the days of less adequate treatment. Hurt (1976) has argued that the attitude adopted by the boy's father is also vital; the most dangerous situation being the one in which the father perceives the boy as a threat to his own image, blames the mother, and rejects the child. The most optimal relationships appear to be those in which both parents provide care, with the mother being most frequently solicitous and the father adopting a more daring attitude to the boy's activities, providing a role model and liberating influence.

While families with a history of hemophilia must be in part prepared for the diagnosis, congenital heart disease has no known similar inherited component. In addition, given the status of the heart in human thought and literature, it is perhaps not surprising that impairments of the heart can take on psychological meaning over and above the physiological implications of the condition. Linde et al. (1966) noted that poorer adjustment and anxiety in the child with a heart condition was more related to maternal anxiety than the degree of incapacity. In turn, maternal anxiety was related to the presence rather than the severity of the condition.

Garson et al. (1978) have listed some questions parents would like answered with regard to congenital heart defect, but which do not tend to be tackled by medical staff. These include the following:

1. Can the particular etiology of the defect be attributed to some action of the mother?
2. Where delays in diagnosis occur, parents are anxious about the implications of delay for prognosis.
3. Parents often are unable to understand physicians' explanations of the diagnosis.
4. Parents are unsure about symptoms to expect; particularly, they may worry as to whether or not a heart attack can occur.
5. Parents may have difficulty explaining the condition to the child.
6. Parents are confused as to how to treat a child with a congenital heart defect normally.

More detailed studies of family coping throughout illness duration have been given by Burton (1975), dealing with cystic fibrosis; Schulman and Kupst (1980), dealing with leukemia; and Koski (1969), dealing with diabetes. For the most part, workers have been content to describe the limitations of an illness and look for general patterns in family coping. More recent work has tried to relate physiological and behavioral measures of the child's illness with aspects of family dynamics. Baker, Rosman, Sargent, and Noguerira (1982), for example, have reported a longitudinal, prospective study of juvenile-onset diabetes. Families were interviewed on diagnosis of diabetes in one of the children. From responses to the questionnaire, the families were evaluated with respect to (1) their ability to support the emotional responses of other family members, (2) their ability to communicate directly with one another, (3) the ability of the parents to adopt different roles without expecting rigid role performance of the other, and (4) joint parental decision making.

Together with the family's affectiveness in controlling the children's behavior during the interview and their effectiveness in getting the sick child to competent medical treatment, these variables correlated with subsequent good control of the child's diabetes.

Disturbed family relations have long been implicated in the so-called psychosomatic disorders, but are now also being implicated in the management of other chronic conditions. According to Minuchin and his co-workers (e.g., Minuchin et al., 1975) a child's symptoms can be viewed as part of the entire family's stress rather than individual stress. Families are perceived as having a role in maintaining the symptom, and in turn, the symptom has a role in stabilizing the family. In one study children with recurrent hospitalizations for unexplained recurrent attacks of asthma or diabetic ketoacidosis were studied. Related work has involved children with hemophilia, sickle cell anemia, inflammatory bowel disease, and juvenile rheumatoid arthritis. Minuchin et al. (1975) identified the following five characteristics in families of children with psychosomatic disorders.

1. *Enmeshment.* This involves extreme interdependence among family members and poor differentiation of members as individual people. The result is extreme sensitivity of family members to each other. Although enmeshment may be appropriate when children are very young, greater distance is required as the children develop. One danger of the enmeshed family is that one parent can enlist the support of one of the children against the other parent.

2. *Overprotectiveness.* Family members have shown an overly high degree of concern for each other. This results in individual incompetence and the inhibition of personal control and problem-solving ability.

3. *Rigidity.* Although these families perceive themselves as normal, they tend to persist with established methods of interaction even where these become inappropriate. Perceptions of the sick child are restricted to the physical problems.

4. *Lack of conflict resolution.* Such families have an especially low tolerance for conflict, and consequently try to avoid conflict wherever possible.

5. *Involvement of the sick child in parental conflict.* Three types of conflict have been noted: *triangulation*, in which the child is expected to side with one or other parent; stable *"parent–child coalition,"* in which the child is always sided with one parent against the other; and *"detouring,"* in which both parents cease their conflicts to protect or attack the sick child.

In the past, little attention has been paid to variables such as these that may influence the course of chronic disease. Yet the variety of responses that have been noted (cf., Pless & Satterwhite, 1975) and our inability to predict the prognosis for many children require that greater attention is paid to these variables in the future.

I have dwelt for some time on "family" reactions to chronic illness in children. This bias, however, has been on parental responses. There is a growing body of literature that suggests that the siblings of a sick child are also affected (for a review see Grave, 1974; Lavigne & Burns, 1981).

Effects of Chronic Illness on Siblings

It is relatively recently that attention has been paid to the emotional and behavioral responses of the siblings of chronically sick children. While children with chronic illness are likely to receive an increased amount of parental and other adult attention, the healthy siblings may find themselves in less advantageous positions. Parents themselves inevitably have less time for their healthy children, especially around times of crisis such as diagnosis. The healthy sibling is likely to be left at short notice with a variety of friends and relations. Outings and other "treats" come to an abrupt end. Healthy children may perceive their own positions in the family to be less than ideal. In part, this can result from parents' inability to inform the sibling of the diagnosis and prognosis for the sick child (Wold & Townes, 1969). Among siblings of children with cystic fibrosis, Turk (1964) noted that these children resented restrictions on their behavior (which included enforced silence and inability to have holidays or friends over to play), but did not fully understand the reasons for these restrictions. In these situations, it is not uncommon for siblings to develop feelings of jealousy and resentment toward the sick child. This can subsequently result in feelings of intense guilt, as the sibling comes to believe that his or her own resentment has precipitated a medical crisis or even death.

These conclusions tend to be based on clinical observations. Often the siblings under study have been referred for psychiatric treatment. As such, their reactions are probably not typical or representative of siblings' general attitudes to a sick brother or sister. Nevertheless, even better controlled studies conclude that the siblings of the chronically sick are at greater risk for the development of behavioral and emotional problems than those with healthy siblings.

Farber (1959, 1960) studied 240 families with a severely mentally retarded child. Siblings younger than the retarded child tended to assume a superordinate role, and female siblings especially were encouraged to adopt a surrogate mother role. These girls showed increased levels of tension, anxiety, and conflict with the natural mother. Female siblings not assigned this care-taking role did not differ from male siblings with regard to conflict with the mother.

Apley, Barbour, and Westmacott (1967) studied siblings of children with congenital heart disease. It was reported that 27% showed some behavior problems, 13% had psychosomatic problems, and 24% had both. Tew, Payne, and Laurence (1974) found that siblings of patients with spina bifida showed a higher incidence of maladjustment than siblings of healthy controls (35% vs. 9%, respectively). McMichael (1971) reported that 21% of healthy siblings showed a moderate or severe degree of failure to adjust in families with a child with a nonfatal physical disorder.

Two studies by Gath (1972, 1973) are also relevant. Gath (1972) studied the 9- to 11-year-old siblings of patients with cleft lip or palate and found no differences between these and siblings of healthy children in frequency of behavior problems. In contrast, Demb and Ruess (cited in Pless & Pinkerton, 1975) noted that, among older siblings of cleft palate patients, the high school dropout rate was higher for siblings (42%) than for the patients (25%) or the general population (30%).

In the second study by Gath (1973), the siblings of 143 children with Down's syndrome were compared with siblings of a matched control group. Parents and teachers completed the relevant scales for behavior problems devised by Rutter and his colleagues. Deviance rates for the two groups were 20% and 10%, respectively, but the main difference between the two groups was in terms of a vastly increased incidence of antisocial behavior among female siblings of the Down's syndrome children. These girls persistently showed signs of difficulty with peer relationships, restlessness, disobedience, misery, and temper tantrums.

Similar findings have been described for siblings of patients with juvenile arthritis. Ivey, Brewer, and Giannini (1981) found that siblings of these patients had higher anxiety levels and lower self-concept than the patients themselves. Miller et al. (1982) also working with juvenile arthritis patients and their siblings asked both groups if they considered themselves limited. Of 50 patients, 5 felt that they were limited, while 8 of 50 siblings reported that they had a chronic illness or disability. Miller et al. suggest that this is consistent with previous findings showing that siblings have higher anxiety levels and lower self-concept than patients with juvenile arthritis.

Some recognition of the difficulties faced by siblings of cancer patients was first acknowledged by Binger (1973). More recently, Powazek, Schyving Payne, Goff, Paulson, and Stagner (1980) reported that 81% of siblings of leukemia patients showed behavior problems during the 1st year following diagnosis.

While it may be true that siblings of sick children are at a greater risk for behavioral and emotional disturbances, there has been little study of variables that might influence their degree of vulnerability. Only one published study appears to attempt to answer this question. Lavigne and Ryan (1979) compared siblings of three groups of patients drawn from hematology, cardiology, and plastic surgery clinics. In addition, there was a control group of healthy children. Younger siblings (aged 3–6 years) of plastic surgery patients showed more behavior problems than children in the other three groups. Among older siblings (aged 7–13 years) there were no differences in incidence of behavior disturbance for any of the comparative groups. In addition, Lavigne and Burns (1981) looked for differences between the groups in terms of specific types of symptoms. The illness groups showed higher levels of social withdrawal and irritability than healthy controls, but did not differ in terms of aggression or learning disability.

A distinction is generally drawn between siblings of children with chronic and those with fatal illnesses. Lavigne and Burns (1981) have summarized the literature concerned with children's reactions to the death of a sibling as follows. First, children exhibit grief responses, ranging from near silence to adult-like expressions of grief including distressed behavior, crying, and talking about the deceased (Bender, cited in Blinder, 1972; Binger, 1973; Cobb, 1956). As Lavigne and Burns note, these expressions of grief are entirely normal, provided they do not continue for excessive periods of time. A second type of response includes emotional or behavioral problems beginning with the sibling's death. In this context, Binger (1973) and Blinder (1972) have noted the onset of somatic complaints; Binger et al. (1969) and Binger (1973) noted depression, and Wold and Townes (1969) noted withdrawal. In addition, several investigators have pointed to academic problems having their onset around the time of death of a sibling (Bender, cited in Blinder, 1972; Binger et al. 1969; Cain, Fast, & Erikson, 1964).

A third type of response includes various distorted behaviors closely related to the death or illness. "Prolonged guilt reactions, suicidal thoughts or the wish to have died instead of the deceased sibling are sometimes noted" (Lavigne & Burns, 1981, p. 347). In the study by Cain et al. (1964), for example, 40% of siblings showed some of the same symptoms as had characterized the illness of the dead brother or sister. Symptoms have been noted to increase around the anniversary of the death. These observations are, however, based on clinical observations. In general it is true to say that there has been little systematic study of the reactions of a child to the death of a sibling. In the few studies that have not confined themselves to clinical populations, it has not been found that such untoward reactions are necessarily the norm. Payne, Goff, and Paulson (1980) found that 36% of children developed academic, psychological, or social problems following the death of a sibling from cancer. Two years later, problems remained for 22%.

Conclusions

The purpose of this chapter has been to provide an overview of research concerned with psychological effects of chronic illness on children and their families. I have tried to identify the most popular research questions and illustrate these with work on a variety of illnesses. In research of this kind, the disease an investigator chooses is determined by a number of factors, many of a practical rather than theoretical nature. Thus, a chronically sick sample is often chosen because there happens to be a center specializing in treatment of this disease near by, or because one consultant is more sympathetic to psychological work than another. For this reason, there have been relatively isolated reports concerned with congenital heart disease, renal disease, or juvenile rheumatoid arthritis, for example. Other illnesses that once warranted research no longer do. These include polio, tuberculosis, or physical disabilities induced by thalidomide. Considerable research effort has been directed at the problems of children with hemophilia, epilepsy, and spina bifida (for reviews see Lindemann, 1981).

The intention of this book is not, however, to be a comprehensive review of all psychological work concerned with chronic illness in childhood. The volume of relevant work is too wide for this to be possible. Rather, the aim is to illustrate the interdependence between the cognitive approach to understanding children's ideas about illness reviewed in Chapter 2, and the applicability of this approach to many of the questions pertinent when dealing with sick children. To do this, I have selected four illnesses as examples, but this is not to say that the approach is not also applicable in other areas. Phenylketonuria is special in many ways, and the research literature somewhat different. The three remaining diseases lend themselves to a more unitary approach. For all three, the research is reviewed under the following headings:

1. Descriptions of the disease and its treatment
2. The effects of the disease on the child (personality factors, children's knowledge about the disease, intellectual development and academic achievement)
3. Effects of the disease on the family

Such an approach hopefully highlights the bias in previous research. Some questions have been extensively researched for one illness, and essentially ignored for another. The classic example is the amount of research effort directed at finding out how much the diabetic child understands about the disease and treatment, while relatively nothing has been published concerned with how the child with asthma understands the illness. By adopting a similar approach to reviewing previous work for each of these illnesses, it is readily apparent where future work needs to be directed.

Part II

Psychological Studies of Specific Chronic Illnesses

5

Phenylketonuria

Before the 1950s the consequences of phenylketonuria (PKU) for the child were quite disastrous. Untreated PKU causes mental retardation; some 96% of patients have IQs below 60 (Baumeister, 1967; Knox, 1960). Surveys of the inmates of institutions suggested that 1 in 100 patients had PKU (Langdell, 1965). In addition to mental retardation, the patient with PKU may suffer from seizures and other neurological abnormalities (Allen & Gibson, 1961; Kang, Kennedy, Gates, Burwash, & McKinnon, 1965). Perceptual motor difficulties (Hackney, Hanley, Davidson, & Lindsao, 1968) and autistic behavior (Lowe, Tanaka, Seashore, Young, & Cohen, 1980) have also been reported.

Causes of the Disease and Treatment

Phenylketonuria is a relatively rare disorder. The incidence has been reported to vary from 1 in 12,000 (Smith & Wolff, 1974) to 1 in 19,000 (Hsia & Holtzman, 1973). Despite the low incidence of the disorder, a great deal of research work has been conducted. Menolascino and Egger (1978) suggest that this is because PKU was the first "inborn error of metabolism" to be discovered that was associated with mental retardation. The hope was that other similar cases of mental retardation would be discovered and that ultimately the incidence of mental retardation in the population could be reduced.

Phenylketonuria was identified by the Norwegian physician Fölling in 1934. The mother of two retarded siblings asked Fölling to treat her children. His account of the subsequent discovery of PKU is impressive.

A mother sought advice because her two children were both mentally retarded. They were 7 and 4 years old, and their unhappy mother had asked for help at many institutions. She had noticed that a peculiar smell always clung to her children. I had no real hope of being able to help her, and I examined the children mainly because I did not want to be hostile to the mother.

By clinical examination of the patients no valuable signs were found, except that the children were definitely feeble-minded. The ordinary urine analyses were also normal, but after adding ferric chloride to the urine a green colour appeared and then disappeared a few minutes later. I had never seen such a reaction and it was not described in the literature. Urine collected a few days later, after withdrawal of all medicants from the patients, behaved similarly. There was probably an unknown substance in the urine, and the first problem seemed to be to isolate and identify this substance. (Bickel, 1980, p. 123)

In subsequent work, Fölling identified eight other cases in local institutions for the mentally retarded and subsequently identified PKU to be inherited as a recessive trait.

In reviewing research into PKU, Bickel (1980) identifies three distinct phases. In the first, between 1934 and 1944, "little more was achieved other than to confirm and amplify Fölling's work from the clinical and genetic point of view" (Bickel, 1980, p. 124). In the following 10 years, considerable advances were made in understanding chemical aspects of PKU. From 1954 to 1964, the most important advance was the development of screening programs to identify PKU soon after birth (Schild, 1979). In the United Kingdom routine neonatal screening was undertaken under the direction of the Medical Research Council (1968), but all western nations now have similar routine screening programs. Komrower (1974) has argued that the costs involved are less than those necessitated by long-term residential care of unidentified individuals.

Phenylketonuria is now classified as an inborn error of protein metabolism. The exact chemistry of the disease is complex, but essentially involves a defect in the conversion of phenylalanine to tyrosine. This results in an excess build-up of amino acid phenyl-alanine, an essential dietary amino acid related to the formation of body protein. Further biochemical, physiological, and pathological effects follow, which contribute to irreversible changes in the central nervous system and hence mental retardation. Differences in severity of the disorder have been noted. In the "classic" form the block in protein synthesis is virtually complete. However, one in six patients have an "atypical" form, in which synthesis is only partially blocked. In these cases, the symptoms are less severe.

Treatment for PKU has changed little since the early 1950s. Children are prescribed diets low in phenylalanine and/or protein. During infancy, children are fed entirely on a synthetic, low phenylalanine formula. Later, children eat foods low in phenylalanine (fruits, vegetables, and cereals). Foods high in phenylalanine (meats, eggs, milk, cheese) are eliminated or restricted. The exact details of foods allowed in low phenylalanine diets vary across treatment centers (Francis, 1975).

Parents shoulder the major responsibility for controlling the child's diet and must become very knowledgeable about food values. They are responsible for keeping food diaries and taking blood samples and urine specimens necessary to monitor the quality of the child's diet. Such monitoring is vital, since there is a real risk of poor physical and mental growth as a result of malnourishment (through low protein intake) rather than a consequence of the disease process itself.

The first case of successful treatment for PKU was reported by Bickel, Gerrard, and Hickmans (1954). They treated a 2-year-old retarded girl by restrictive diet, and reported an improvement in both behavior and general development. Subsequent work has indicated that introduction of the diet before 3 months of age is essential in order to facilitate normal mental development.

Effects of Phenylketonuria on the Child

Research effort has shifted from a climate in which the question was one of when the diet should be introduced to reduce the degree of retardation, to one of when it may be discontinued. The blandness of the diet makes it very unappetizing, and older children especially are likely to rebel. The tension created during mealtimes prompted many families to press for a complete or partial relaxation of the diet as soon as possible. Treatment centers still vary, however, in when they believe it is safe for a child to adopt a normal diet.

Early work was consistent in suggesting that early introduction of the diet (before 2 months of age) was essential for normal mental growth (Hudson, Mordaunt, & Leahy, 1970; Schmid-Rüter & Grubel-Kaiser, 1977). As a general rule, introduction of the diet after 1 year of age is less successful.

Although early introduction of the diet is apparently associated with near-normal levels of intelligence, treated children with PKU still tend to score below other family members on IQ tests (cf., Berman, Graham, Eichman, & Waisman, 1961; Berman, Waisman, & Graham, 1966; Centrewall & Centrewall, 1961; Dobson, Williamson, Azen, & Koch, 1977; Smith, Lobascher, & Wolff, 1973; Smith & Wolff, 1974; Woolf, Griffiths, Moncrieff, Coates, & Dillistone, 1958).

Hsia (1967) reported that patients' IQ scores, even after introduction of the diet within the first 2 months, were 24 points below those of unaffected siblings. Despite early treatment, these authors reported that patients were less intelligent than unaffected siblings. Berman et al.

(1961), for example, investigated eight children, five of whom were placed on appropriate diets before 3 months of age. Treated children scored better than untreated siblings, but lower than unaffected siblings. If the level of functioning shown by unaffected siblings is assumed to indicate the best level that might be achieved by a treated child, the implications must be that even early initiated diet is not necessarily compatible with optimal intellectual functioning.

A larger scale study was reported by Berman et al. (1966), in which 22 treated children were compared with their 50 siblings. By assessing serum phenylalanine levels of the siblings, it was found that six had untreated phenylketonuria. The children were assessed over a 27-month period. At both the beginning and the end of this study, treated PKU children had lower IQ scores than unaffected siblings. They report that a subgroup of eight patients treated before 4 months of age had a mean IQ score of 27.5 points below unaffected siblings. Gains in IQ scores between first and last testing sessions were made by all children except for the unaffected siblings, suggesting some cumulative beneficial effects of the diet. Nevertheless, the size of the differences between treated children and unaffected family members is indeed very large.

Smith et al. (1973) studied a group of PKU children treated from early infancy, and where possible, compared their IQ scores with unaffected siblings and parents. Eight patients were found to have a mean IQ score of 89, significantly below that of their eight unaffected siblings (mean = 110.25). Smith et al. report that a correlation in IQ scores of +0.53 is found between siblings in the normal population, yet there is no such correlation between PKU children and their siblings. The authors were also able to assess the mothers of 17 PKU children and the fathers of 12. The mean score for mothers and fathers was 100.5. Again this score showed no correlation with the IQ scores of the PKU children. It is regrettable that authors do not tend to report the correlation in IQ scores between parents and unaffected as well as affected children, since it would be useful to know if this differed at all from that of the normal population. Although a child's IQ is normally correlated with father's occupation, there was again no correlation between IQ of PKU children and father's occupation. The implications of this series of results is that normal environmental correlates of intelligence between family members are lacking in affected PKU children, suggesting that apparently adequate dietary treatment, even when initiated early in life, is not able to overcome completely the biological limitations of the condition.

In their study concerned with the effects of early treatment on intelligence in PKU, Smith and Wolff (1974) investigated 28 PKU children and their siblings. In some cases the sibling being born after an older child had already been identified as having PKU was placed on an appropriate diet in the neonatal period. These children all had IQ scores above 70. Children who were identified beyond the neonatal period had IQ scores in the range of 30–37.

Dobson et al. (1977) assessed 203 children at 4 years of age who had begun diet therapy between 3 and 92 days after birth. The mean Stanford-Binet IQ of the group (93) was 12 and 17 points below the mean for the mothers and fathers, respectively.

Berry, O'Grady, Perlmutter, and Bofinger (1979) investigated IQ of children with PKU in relation to both unaffected siblings and parents. Twenty children beginning diet early in infancy (mean age on beginning diet = 16.4 days) still had IQ scores significantly lower than those of their parents or siblings (mean IQ of patients = 98; mothers = 110.2; fathers = 116.1; and unaffected siblings = 107.2). Six late-treated children scored even worse in relation to other family members (mean IQ of late-treated group = 50.8; mothers = 116; fathers = 122; and unaffected siblings = 103.8).

Several hypotheses have been advanced as to why treated children continue to show deficits in relation to unaffected family members. The most favored explanation suggests that poor dietary control is responsible (McBean & Stephenson, 1968). Supporting this argument, Sutherland, Hudson, and Hawcroft (1978) have reported an inverse relationship between IQ at 4 years and mean phenylalanine concentration during the child's 4th year, i.e., lower IQ is associated with a less well-controlled child. An alternative hypothesis is that delay in diagnosis accounts for the discrepancy, and certainly there are several studies that suggest that improved intellectual functioning is associated with earlier initiation of diet (e.g., Berry, et al. 1979; Kang, Sallee, and Gerald, 1970; Smith & Wolff, 1974). In view of the difficulty in balancing the diet, Hanley, Linsao, Davidson, & Moes (1970) have suggested that malnutrition is the cause of some intellectual loss. An alternative explanation by Saugstad (1972) is that the reduced intellectual functioning is due to residual prenatal damage.

Additional work has suggested that children with PKU underfunction in other areas of development. Reports of learning difficulties (Leonard, Chase, & Childs (1972), behavior problems (Stevenson et al., 1979), perceptual–motor disabilities (Koff, Boyle, & Pueschel, 1977), lowered self-esteem (Moen, Wilcox, & Burns, 1977), and language disabilities (Melnick, Michaels, & Matalon, 1981) have been made.

Linguistic Development

Early studies of general development in PKU were suggestive of some delay in speech and language abilities (cf., Berry et al. 1979). Other more systematic studies of language (Koch et al., 1973) were restricted to children of 5–7 years. Little, therefore, is known about the process of early language acquisition in these children. However, Melnick et al. (1981) studied the language development of 12 early treated children with PKU, all of normal intelligence. The children were aged between 4 and 62 months and were assessed over a period of 7 to 33 months. On a

quite extensive battery of language tests, six of the children were found
to be developing normally, and six showed language delay. The authors
concluded that even children with normal intelligence and PKU show a
greater predominance of language disabilities than the normal population. The data in fact suggest that the incidence of language problems
could be greater than the authors suggest, since those children
described as most normal in language skills were also the youngest, (i.e.,
children aged 4, 5, 9, and 10 months on initial testing).

Apparently contradictory results to these have been made in a
preliminary report by Zartler and Sassaman (1981). Children between 2
and 6 years of age were studied, and Zartler and Sassaman report that
most children showed language development to be at a similar rate to
general cognitive development. None of the children were ever thought
to need additional speech therapy. Although these authors conclude
that PKU children do not show language deficits, they acknowledge that
further study is needed. They also report that children did show deficits
in perceptual–motor and arithmetic skills.

Behavior

Stevenson et al. (1979) surveyed the behavior of 99 early treated PKU
children. When the children were 8-years-old, parents were asked to
complete the Rutter behavior questionnaire "A" (Rutter, Tizard, &
Whitmore, 1970), and teachers completed the corresponding scale "B"
(Rutter, 1967).

> The Rutter parent and teacher scales consist of descriptions of behaviour
> rated as "certainly applies", "applies somewhat" and "doesn't apply"
> (scored 2, 1, and 0 respectively). The teacher scale has 26 such items and the
> parent scale 18; the parent scale has, in addition, 13 items on health and
> habits (similarly scored 2, 1, and 0). Children scoring 9 or more on the
> teacher scale or 13 or more on the parent scale, have been shown by Rutter
> to have a higher risk of psychiatric disorder than those with lower scores.
> Furthermore, the deviant behaviour shown by children with high scores
> can be classified into 3 diagnostic types—antisocial, neurotic, or mixed—
> depending on the ratings of relevant individual items. (Stevenson et al.,
> 1979, p. 15)

In addition, teachers completed the same questionnaire for two other
children in the class. The IQ data were available for 86 of the PKU
children. Significantly more of the PKU children showed behavior
deviance on the teacher scale compared with the "control" children
(40% vs. 20%, respectively). More of the PKU children showed neurotic
behavior (22% vs. 8%), but there was no significant difference between
the groups in antisocial deviance. Parents identified fewer of the
children as deviant than teachers, but like teachers, they were more
likely to identify neurotic than antisocial deviance.

Stevenson et al. (1979) point out that the 40% rate of behavior deviance identified by teachers of PKU children is higher than the rate identified for any other investigated group. They hypothesize that this result may be attributable to (1) a direct effect of raised blood phenylalanine levels on brain cell metabolism; (2) effects of phenylalanine on brain development in early life; (3) psychological effects of abnormal diet directly on the child or via disturbed family relationships; and (4) a genetic mechanism whereby the gene responsible for PKU also produces a vulnerability to psychiatric disturbance.

The findings should be contrasted to those of Siegel, Barlow, Fisch, and Anderson (1968). Using an unstandardized school behavior profile, Siegel et al. compared 13 PKU children with normal controls. No differences between the groups were found. However, the numbers of children involved were small, and the questionnaire of doubtful reliability. The very significant levels of disturbance found by Stevenson et al. (1979) suggests that their data are not simply due to chance.

Diet Termination in Phenylketonuria

It was initially hoped that PKU was a childhood problem and that the diet need only be maintained during the preschool years, by which time the brain in effectively fully developed (Vandeman, 1963). Despite these early claims, much controversy still surrounds the issue of when, if at all, the diet can safety be terminated. Deterioration in both intelligence and behavior have been reported for children beginning normal diets.

A recent review by Waisbren, Schnell, and Levy (1980) summarized work published prior to 1979. Of these 19 papers, all used intelligence tests as the basic assessment of the effectiveness of the diet. "Of these 19 studies, nine (288 subjects) reported a substantial IQ loss for some of the children, and ten (123 subjects) reported either no negative consequences or only slight trends in a negative direction" (Waisbren et al., 1980, p. 149). Some of the earlier studies may be dismissed because of poor procedures and controls. The following studies have been selected for more detailed descriptions, since they involve an acceptable sample size and reasonable attempts at methodological control.

Cabalska, Duczynska, Borzymowska, Zorska, Koślacz-Folga, & Bozkowa (1977) investigated three groups of patients. Twenty-two children showed classic PKU with a mean treatment period of 4 years 8 months; 10 showed cases of classic PKU with a mean treatment of 2 years 4 months and 5 showed cases of variant PKU with a mean treatment period of 3 years 8 months. All children were followed for 4- 6 years after diet termination. Assessments of mental development, clinical symptoms, behavior, school achievements, and electroencephalogram (EEG) ratings were made. Among the children with classic PKU, decreases in intelligence were found following diet termination. These patients also showed difficulties in school achievements and behavior, as well as abnormalities in EEG patterns. In contrast, patients with PKU variants did not show corresponding declines in intelligence or behavior. Cabalska et al. therefore argued that cases of classic PKU require treatment for more than the first 5 years of life.

One problem in interpreting some of these data is that many children of school age place themselves on relaxed diets, so that phenylalanine levels are poorly controlled in the period immediately before diet termination. Their IQ scores and behavior may then be artificially low when they are believed to be on well-controlled diets, and this would result in apparently no adverse effects of stopping treatment. A relaxed diet, which was acceptable to the child and family and sufficient to arrest mental deterioration, could have advantages over a normal diet, but not be associated with adverse behavioral and intellectual signs. A comparison between two such diets has been reported by Smith et al. (1978). They compared 47 children treated at the Hospital for Sick Children, London, England, who were placed on a normal diet when aged between 5 and 15 years of age, with 22 patients treated in Heidelberg, Germany, who were placed on relaxed phenylalanine diets. For both centers the data were analyzed separately for children who began controlled diets early (mean age = 6 weeks) and those beginning controlled diets when older (mean age = just under 2 years). Between the last IQ test on strict diet and the IQ measured at intervals of 1, 2, and 3 years after diet change, there were consistent falls in IQ score for all groups. Patients in London on normal diets showed reductions in IQ of 5 to 9 points, while patients in Heidelberg on relaxed diets showed somewhat smaller losses in IQ. In addition, there was a suggestion that children who changed diets after 9 years of age showed smaller losses in IQ than those changing before 9 years. These data suggest that even for children placed on an appropriate diet before 6 weeks of age, it would be unwise even to relax the diet before the child is 9 years old.

The study by Smith et al. (1978) can be criticized on several grounds. Studies of this kind need to include a control group of patients on strict diet if they are to be readily interpreted. In the study by Smith et al. (1978), families were allowed to decide for themselves when to change diet. Factors influencing a family to give up strict diet may in themselves be associated with reductions in IQ. Accurate assessments of the effects of diet termination can thus only be made by systematically assigning families to conditions in which diets must be strictly maintained, relaxed, or terminated. In the United States PKU Collaborative Project, 22% of parents refused to be allocated randomly to such conditions (Williamson, Koch, & Berlow, 1979). Fifteen treatment centers together conducted a randomized trial of the effects of stopping diet involving 140 children. All children began treatment in the neonatal period, and at age 6 years were randomly assigned to terminate or continue on strict diet. It was at this stage that 22% of parents refused to take part. One year after diet change, 83 children were assessed, and of these, 55 were reassessed 2 years later. In children who continued on diet, there was a slight rise in IQ (mean IQ at 6 years = 97, at 8 years = 101). Children taken off the diet showed a deterioration over the same period (mean IQ at 6 years = 97, at 7 years = 96; at 8 years = 91).

Taken together, these results suggest that although some children do not appear to be adversely affected by stopping diet, others show slight or sometimes more substantial losses in IQ. The confusion in the literature has led some authors to argue that the research question needs to be changed (Lindeman, 1981; Waisbren et al., 1980). For the future the concern need not be with *when* phenylalanine-controlled diets can be terminated, but rather with describing those individuals who can safely terminate diet and those who need to remain under more strict dietary control. The study by Cabalska et al. (1977), in distinguishing between the variants of PKU, represents a first attempt to do this.

However, even these conclusions seem inadequate, given a study by Brunner, Jordon, and Berry (1983) in which children's performance on a number of neuropsychological measures was inversely related to serum phenylalanine levels. Brunner et al. compared 27 children with PKU, diagnosed and placed on appropriate diets since infancy, with unaffected siblings and age-matched nonfamilial controls. There were significant differences between the groups in measured intelligence, school achievement, concept formation and tactile–motor problem solving. Serum phenylalanine concentration on the day of neuro-psychological testing was negatively correlated with performance. These results may be interpreted as evidence that even slight increases in phenylalanine levels resulting from terminating strict diet may be inadvisable.

Effects of Phenylketonuria on the Family

The diet creates many difficulties for the family. Parents must learn the intricacies of the disease, diet, and its monitoring. In particular, they must learn to prepare special meals and integrate them into the family's menu. Everyday arguments about foods between parent and child, which are experienced by all families, take on a new meaning where parents are anxious that food refusal may lead to mental retardation. Eating away from home, at school, in restaurants, or at birthday parties require special planning. Acosta, Fiedler, and Koch (1968) reported a questionnaire study designed to describe special problems experienced by families with a PKU child. Forty-seven families completed a postal questionnaire. (Seventy-four questionnaires were posted originally.) Although 63% of mothers who replied said they had no difficulties in preparing the child's food, 20% reported difficulties. These included "incorporation of color and variety in a menu based on the child's limited food preferences, seemingly inadequate portions and the bareness of the child's plate, and the need for consistently serving very simple foods" (Acosta et al., 1968, p. 461). Despite the fact that 84% of the children involved were of an age when they could eat food from the family's meals, only 57% of mothers actually permitted this, 24% occasionally fed the child the same as the rest of the family, and 8% of mothers always prepared a special meal for the PKU child. Forty-three percent of mothers stated that there were some feeding problems with the child. Given the restrictive nature of the diet, it is small wonder that many parents pressure medical staff to agree to allow the child a normal diet as soon as possible.

Conclusions

This chapter has briefly described some of the contributions made by psychologists to the care and treatment of children with PKU. As in the management of other chronic conditions, there remains room for considerable additional work. Little is known about the impact of PKU on family life. Parental understanding of the disease has been reported to be poor or distorted (Fisch, Conley, Eysenbach, & Chang, 1977; Keleske, Solomon, & Opitz, 1967; Wood, Friedman, & Steisel, 1967). At the same time, the question of how the children themselves understand their condition is essentially unresearched. As PKU is diagnosed in the newborn period, education about the disease is naturally directed at the parents. It needs to be acknowledged that the children also require an explanation as they grow older. Education of the children may result in greater compliance with the diet and treatment. Whether it has this effect or not, education is also necessary for girls of childbearing age. There is a real risk that PKU can be transmitted to the offspring (Komrower, Saroharwalla, Coutts, & Ingham, 1979). Reintroduction of the diet, *prior to conception*, appears the only way to safeguard the health of the next generation (Buist, Lis, Tuerck, & Murphy, 1979; Komrower et al., 1979). Girls with PKU therefore need to be taught about the potential risk for their children and undertake to place themselves on restrictive diets before they conceive.

There have been few attempts to describe how parents perceive or interact with their PKU children. Implications of work with handicapped groups suggest that such interactions are affected by parental feelings of guilt. In that PKU has a hereditary component, it is natural that some parents will experience feelings of guilt and self-blame for the child's condition. Both Johnson (1979) and Schild (1979) have reported that parents of PKU children have strong feelings of guilt, anxiety, and frustration, and that these color qualitative aspects of parent–child interaction and decisions about child rearing generally.

Instead, attempts to describe the impact of PKU on family life have tended to focus on management of the diet (Wood et al., 1967). Acosta et al. (1968) concluded that advice to parents was especially needed in the areas of menu planning, food preparation, feeding problems, discipline, and normal child growth and development. Parental difficulties in maintaining children on this diet have led to a demand to terminate the diet as soon as possible. Assessments of the feasibility of this have been based on IQ scores of the children while on and off the diet. Decisions about diet termination should not, however, be based on IQ data alone. For this reason, some attempts to consider emotional well-being (Bentovim, 1968; Chang & Fisch, 1976; Goldstein & Frankenberg, 1970; Pueschel, Yeatman, & Hum, 1977); visual motor coordination (Donker et al., 1978; Rolle-Daya, Pueschel, & Lombrosco, 1975); and EEG patterns (Chang & Fisch, 1976; Koff et al., 1977; Parker, 1973; Siegel et al., 1968) have been made. Unfortunately, decisions about dietary management still tend to be made on the basis of IQ information alone. The onus is on psychologists to develop reliable tests of attention and cognition that are as acceptable to other professionals as are IQ measures.

6

Diabetes

There is probably no other disease in which psychology is as relevant as in diabetes. The pediatrician must secure the cooperation of the child and parents in order to maximize compliance to medical care and minimize the incidence of poor control and long-term complications. Traditionally, psychologists have been concerned with identifying a "diabetic personality." This research is reviewed briefly, and its shortcomings noted. The emphasis in this chapter is on how the child understands the disease and its implications at different ages, and the relevance of these data in communicating with the sick child. In this respect, the review is organized around (1) the child's general information about diabetes, (2) the child's beliefs about how diabetes affects the body, and (3) the child's awareness of future complications.

In addition to this emphasis on knowledge, there is a second area in which psychology is relevant. As with other chronic diseases, the potential damage that a diagnosis of diabetes might have for the family is considerable. Specific research into family functioning in diabetes is reviewed.

Diabetes is one of the more "acceptable" of the chronic conditions. Abroms and Kodera (1979), for example, asked healthy college students to rank 15 disabling conditions in terms of personal acceptability. Diabetes was ranked third after ulcers and asthma. A study by Davis, Shipp, and Pattishall (1965) similarly reports that children with diabetes did not wish to trade their disease for a less life-threatening but more visible problem, such as obesity. All the children in this study stated that they would prefer to have diabetes rather than constipation, and a high percentage apparently would rather have diabetes than a pimple or six toes! Notwithstanding these results, the potential threat that diabetes poses to the child's social, intellectual, and physical development should not be underestimated.

Indeed, where children were given a choice between freedom from diabetes and other presumably desirable things, such as having more money, being better looking, playing games better, being smarter, and having more friends, the majority chose freedom from their diabetes (Thompson, Garner, & Partridge, 1969).

Diabetes is one of the more common chronic conditions, affecting 1.43 per 1,000 children (Calnan & Peckham, 1977). There is some evidence also that prevalence of the condition is increasing (Stewart-Brown, Haslum, & Butler, 1983).

Causes of the Disease and Treatment

Diabetes is a metabolic disorder of unknown origin. Failure of the pancreas to produce insulin prevents the body from utilizing carbo-hydrates for energy. Consequently, sugar is lost as a fuel, spills into the blood and then to the urine. It is thought that this failure of the pancreas may be caused by a number of factors. Diabetes can be inherited through a recessive gene, but it seems that what is inherited is not diabetes as such, but the predisposition for the disease to develop under the influence of environmental agents (Johnston & Tattersall, 1981). Current thinking suggests that a virus may be responsible. Peak incidences of diabetes occur at 5 and 11 years of age. Children tend to begin or change school at this age and may therefore be exposed to a new set of viruses. This is often quoted as support for the virus theory.

The most pervasive evidence that diabetes does not have a single cause comes from the fact that *juvenile-onset* diabetes, developing before 15 years of age, is very different from *maturity-onset* diabetes. In the juvenile form the pancreas produces no insulin at all, and the disease must be controlled by insulin injections. The mature form is less severe; the pancreas produces some insulin, and the disease can be controlled by diet and pills alone.

In the diabetic the normal process involving the metabolism of sugar to energy breaks down. Starchy foods are broken down to glucose in the normal way, but absence of insulin results in glucose remaining in the bloodstream until the kidneys are reached. Since there is so much glucose, the kidneys are unable to extract the glucose and therefore it is excreted in the urine. Since glucose carries water with it, a symptom of diabetes is excessive passing of urine (*polyuria*). This leads to the second symptom, excessive thirst (*polydipsia*). Finally, as the body is not being fueled by glucose, it must rely for energy on previously stored fat. This leads to the final symptom, excess eating (*polyphagia*). The result is, nevertheless, weight loss.

In the acute stage the child may present with severe abdominal pain and may go into coma, *ketoacidosis*. Diabetes is controlled by the injection of insulin to counter the body's inability to produce its own. It is necessary however, to adjust the amount of insulin injected according to the body's needs, and these may be influenced by factors such as exercise, anxiety, or illness. The child with diabetes or a parent must learn to test the sugar content of the child's urine and blood, adjust the insulin dose, and inject appropriately.

Diabetics are usually advised in addition to adopt recommended diets. Some authorities favor a relatively "free" diet, recommending the use of polyunsaturated fats, the avoidance of concentrated sweets, and a regular pattern of food intake. Others are more insistent on very organized and restrictive diets with carefully calculated weights of carbohydrates, proteins, and fats (Ehrlich, 1974). Between these two extremes are a range of recommended positions. Nuttall (1983) has reviewed the research into the role of diet in prevention of long-term complications of diabetes, and concludes that there is little scientific evidence for the value of strict dietary control. More recently, a number of physicians have recommended a "high-fiber" diet (Miranda & Horwitz, 1978) and claim that this is successful in helping control diabetes, without requiring careful weighing of foods as in traditional carbohydrate exchange programs.

After diagnosis, the patient must expect some major changes in life-style. Regular urine testing and blood monitoring becomes necessary to estimate the level of sugar in the body. As a result of these tests, the child or parent must determine the appropriate levels of insulin needed and prepare and administer the injection. It is unfortunately true that long-term complications occur with diabetes, and these become more frequent the longer the patient has the disease. Individuals developing diabetes during childhood are therefore especially at risk. Three systems of the body are susceptible: the vascular, the retinal, and the neural systems (Kohrman & Weil, 1971; Paulsen & Colle, 1969).

There have been several attempts to describe which aspects of diabetes and its treatment are most distressing to patients. Frish, Galatzer, & Laron (1977) found that injections were generally reported to be the "worst" thing about diabetes, while Fallstrom (1974) found that "anxiety about future complications" was the worst. Galatzer, Frish, and Laron (1977) looked at changes in the "degree of bothersomeness" reported by a group of 30 young diabetics. These patients were first interviewed in 1966 and again in 1975 and were asked to rank 10 aspects of diabetes in order of "bothersomeness", with 1 being the most bothersome and 10, the least. Injections were ranked first on each occasion. Other results are shown in Table 6-1. As part of a larger study,

Table 6-1. Degree of Bothersomeness for Aspects of Diabetes Ranked by 30 Diabetics

Aspects	Rank in 1966	Rank in 1975
Injections	1	1
Hypo[glycemic attack]	2	3
Fear of future limitations in occupations	3	6
Feeling different from others	4	10
Diabetic limitations	5	4
Future complications	6	2
Meals	7	5
Daily urine samples	8	7
Fear that others know	9	9
Having to record urine results	10	8

Note: 1 = most bothersome; 10 = least bothersome.
Note. From "Changes in self-concept and feelings towards diabetic adolescents" by A. Galatzer, M. Frish, and Z. Laron. In Z. Laron (Ed.) *Pediatric adolescent endocrinology: Vol. 3. Psychological aspects of balance of diabetes in juveniles*, 1977, Basel: Karger. Reprinted by permission.

Eiser, Patterson, and Town (in press) asked 57 diabetic children what they thought was the "worst" thing about diabetes. As reported by Frish et al. (1977) and Galatzer et al. (1977), "injections" were considered to be the worst thing by a majority (56.1%). In addition, children objected to the "tests" (29.9%), the restrictions placed on diet (21.1%), and hospital visits (29.8%).

Effects of Diabetes on the Child

Personality Factors in Diabetes

Previous reviews have differed in their organization of the research literature. S. B. Johnson (1980) for example, identified three main research issues: (1) the influence of psychosocial factors on the onset of diabetes, (2) the influence of psychosocial factors on the course of the disease, and (3) the influence of diabetes on the psychosocial development of the child. Garner and Thompson (1974b) identified five issues: (1) the interdependence of metabolic disorder and emotional behavior, (2) the impact of diabetes on the usual stages of development, (3) the ways in which the clinical characteristics of diabetes affect the child and family, (4) reactions to the therapeutic regimen, and (5) the methods that children and families adopt to cope with the condition.

It has traditionally been hypothesized that diabetes has a psychological component. During the seventeenth century Willis suggested that the disease was the result of a "long sorrow." There is increasing evidence of some link between stress and illness (cf., Coddington, 1972; Holmes & Rahe, 1967), and diabetes is no exception to this general statement. Stein and Charles (1971) studied 38 child and adolescent patients, and the authors reported a higher incidence of parental loss and severe family disturbance than in a matched group of non-diabetic patients. These results have not gone uncriticized. S. B. Johnson (1980) for example, has argued that some of the stress did in fact occur 6–10 years prior to the onset of diabetes, a time period possibly too long past to be of any significance. Further, the patients in the Stein and Charles study were primarily of lower socioeconomic status, and it is unclear how representative of the general population they might be. The findings were based on patient's recall of significant events, and these may well have been colored by the patient's illness experiences. Johnson also suggests that the data may reflect the fact that Stein and Charles were fairly convinced of the association between diabetes-onset and previous life stress. Thus, no attempt was made to ensure that raters were unaware of whether the child was in the diabetic or comparison group. Other investigators have suggested that parents may prefer to point to a distressing event occurring prior to disease-onset, rather than recognize the role of hereditary factors (Frankel, 1975; Laron, Karp, & Frankel, 1972). Especially during the 1950s, however, much research was channeled into a search for the "diabetic personality"; an attempt to describe a group of personality traits that might predispose an individual to develop diabetes. Dunbar (1954), for example, described the typical diabetic as showing dependence–independence conflicts, poor sexual adjustment, anxiety, and paranoid depression. Many later workers have also argued that there is a higher incidence of emotional and behavioral disorders among diabetics than normals (Katz, 1957; Swift, Seidman, & Stein, 1967).

This approach is, however, very much in disrepute. Even if a difference in personality traits were discovered between diabetics and normals, it is rarely possible to be certain if this occurred prior to the onset of diabetes or as a result of the disease. We should not really be surprised if an individual with a potentially life-threatening and certainly life-long disease is more anxious or dependent than healthy counterparts. Yet this is as far as much early research goes. Groups of diabetics were asked to complete paper-and-pencil assessments of such traits as anxiety, hostility, or aggression, and the responses were compared with "matched" control groups. The findings were singularly inconsistent. Using a projective measure of anxiety, Fallstrom (1974) reported that diabetics were especially anxious. However, these data were not replicated by Appelboom-Fondu, Verstraeten, and Van Loo-Reynaers (1977); McCraw and Tuma (1977); or Sayed and Leaverton (1974). Using more objective measures, Tavormina, Kastner, Slater, and Watt (1976) and Steinhauser, Borner, and Koepp (1977) also reported that diabetics were not highly anxious. There have been equally confused results where investigators have looked at hostility or aggression in the diabetic patient (Appelboom-Fondu et al., 1977; Fallstrom, 1974; McCraw & Tuma, 1977; Sayed & Leaverton, 1974).

More consistent evidence exists that diabetics do have difficulties in peer relationships and social adjustment (Delbridge, 1975; Fallstrom, 1974; Sayed & Leaverton, 1974; Tavormina et al., 1976). Other work suggests that diabetic children may suffer from a lowering of self-esteem and negative self-image (Richardson, Hastorf, & Dornbusch, 1964; Swift et al., 1967). Sullivan (1979) asked 100 adolescent girls to complete a scale of self-esteem, a Diabetes Adjustment Scale, and depression inventory. Girls with lower self-esteem scored lower in terms of overall adjustment and had difficulties with peer and family relationships. Girls with lower adjustment scores were more depressed. Bruhn (1977) has described how diabetes can adversely influence an individual's self-concept. Bruhn suggests that the reactions of the family and way in which the physician informs the patient about the condition and its treatment are critical determinants of how an individual's self-concept may be compromised.

The role of self-image or self-concept in determining the adjustment of any chronically sick person has appeal at both an intuitive and theoretical level. Yet there is much research work to be done, particularly in clarifying the definitions of these concepts and identifying the mechanisms at work, before this type of research can expect to gain any real status (Lavigne & Burns, 1981).

One personality dimension of potential importance especially to children with diabetes is *locus of control*. The internal–external control of reinforcement (I–E) is an expectancy variable referring to the extent that an individual perceives that what happens is dependent on personal action as opposed to chance, luck, or fate. It is of special relevance in diabetes, since so much of the management of the disease is dependent on the patient's own behavior.

The potential researcher has a degree of choice in selecting an instrument to measure locus of control in children. Many opt for one of the well-established scales devised to measure generalized beliefs among children, such as the scale by Nowicki and Strickland (1973), the Nowicki-Strickland Children's Locus of Control, (NSCLC), or Bialer-Cromwell, (Bialer, 1961). The NSCLC for example, is a 40-item forced-choice questionnaire that can be group administered. The items describe "reinforcement situations which include interpersonal and motivational areas such as affiliation, achievement, and dependency" (Eggland, 1973, p. 311). Typical items include the following:

1. Are some kids just born lucky?
2. Most of the time, do you feel that you can change what might happen tomorrow by what you do today?
3. Do you think that kids can get their own way if they just keep trying?

The need to develop specific scales to measure specific categories of behavior has been repeatedly emphasized (Lefcourt, 1972; Rotter, 1975) and resulted in a scale to measure health locus of control beliefs among adults (Wallston, Wallston, Kaplan, & Maides, 1976). As regard to health, it has been argued that "internals, in contrast to externals, would be more sensitive to health messages, would have increased knowledge about health conditions, would attempt to improve physical functioning, and might even, through their own efforts, be less susceptible to physical and psychological dysfunction" (Strickland, 1978, p. 1193).

Acknowledging the potential importance of health locus of control beliefs, especially in educating children about health, Parcel and Meyer (1978) developed a 20-item forced-choice questionnaire. Examples of this scale include the following:

1) Good health comes from being lucky.
2) It is my mother's job to keep me from getting sick.
3) Accidents just happen.
4) I can make many choices about my health.
5) There is nothing I can do to have healthy teeth. (p. 154)

Factor analyses conducted by Parcel and Meyer (1978) yielded the following three factors:

1. (P) powerful others control subscale
2. (I) internal control subscale
3. (C) chance control subscale

While Parcel and Meyer (1978) reported a significant but not high correlation between the Children's Health Locus of Control (CHLC) scale and the NSCLC scale, no data regarding the predictability of the CHLC for children's behavior are available. There remain problems in the design and validity of both scales. This has not, however, deterred researchers from investigating children's locus of control beliefs in many situations. With regard to chronic illness, two main questions can be identified:

1. Does the experience of chronic illness influence an individual's locus of control beliefs? In particular, it has been predicted that chronic illness and its accompanying reduction in independence and self-

sufficiency may lead to more external beliefs than among healthy individuals.

2. How do individual locus of control beliefs influence adjustment to the disease? It might be predicted, for example, that internals would learn more about their diseases, and adopt more "compliant" attitudes and behaviors than their sick, externally oriented counterparts.

The literature regarding locus of control beliefs among adults has been extensively reviewed (Strickland, 1978; Wallston & Wallston, 1978; Wallston & Wallston, 1981). Considering only the literature on pediatric patients, there is some evidence that chronic illness or handicap is associated with more external locus of control beliefs. Land and Vineberg (1965) studied 27 children made blind before 5 years of age and 27 healthy controls. The blind children had significantly more external beliefs than the healthy children. Similar results were obtained by Eggland (1973) comparing children with cerebral palsy and a group of nonhandicapped. Other results have not necessarily been consistent with these data. Bruhn, Hampton, and Chandler (1971) reported that hemophiliacs were more internal in their beliefs than normals.

Some of these inconsistencies may be resolved by considering the degree to which any one illness limits a child's potential for normal functioning. While it is true that many illnesses do make a child more dependent on others for help and care, other illnesses are much more under individual control. This applies for example, to the ability of a hemophiliac to control bleeding episodes (Agle, 1964; Lucas, 1965; Steinhausen, 1975). An individual's locus of control orientation has therefore been considered as crucial in understanding differences between individuals in the extent to which they are prepared to learn about, or take responsibility for, their own disease. Several recent reports concerned with diabetic patients offer some support for these arguments. Working with adults, Goldstein (1980) found that those with better con trolled diabetes did hold more internal beliefs. Lowery and Ducette (1976) reported that adults with internal locus of control beliefs acquired knowledge of the disease more quickly than those with external beliefs, and Alogna (1980) found that compliant adult patients had more internal locus of control beliefs than noncompliant patients. Compliant patients also tended to be older and to perceive their disease as more serious than the noncompliant.

Locus of control among pediatric diabetic patients has been investigated by Moffatt and Pless (1983). One hundred and fifty-six children were administered both the NSCLC and the CHLC at the beginning and end of a 3-week diabetics camp. At the beginning of camp, the children were also rated in terms of the overall adjustment to the disease. Ratings of diabetes control and knowledge were made by two physicians, ratings of self-help technical skill by two nurses, ratings of diet knowledge and adherence by two dieticians, and ratings of adjustment to camp life by two camp staff members. These ratings were highly related to locus of control beliefs at the beginning of camp, i.e., well-adjusted children had more internal beliefs.

At the end of the 3-week camp experience, it was found that locus of control beliefs for the children shifted in the direction of increased internality at least as measured by the NSCLC. No change was recorded on the CHLC. A subsample of children were assessed 1 year later and continued to show internal locus of control beliefs on the NSCLC. Moffatt and Pless (1983) argue that an internal belief orientation is desirable among diabetics. Certainly most physicians would argue that the relationship between diabetes self-management and biological control is likely to be enhanced by patient's belief of self-control. There was however, no attempt to identify what aspect of the camp experience influenced the children. Whether internal beliefs were fostered simply by being with other diabetic children or by the information children received while at camp is open to question. At a theoretical level, there was no attempt to explain why a shift in beliefs was picked up on the CHLC scale but not according to the NSCLC scale. These data suggest, however, that locus of control beliefs may be critical in determining an individual's reaction to diabetes if not to all chronic illnesses.

Children's Knowledge About Diabetes

General Information About Diabetes

Probably more than any other condition, diabetes demands that patients are as responsible for their own care as the physician. For this reason, much research has been directed at ascertaining how much information children have about the disease, its cause, and treatment. On the basis of this work, there have been attempts to recommend suitable chronological ages at which it is felt that children would be capable of self-care.

Some of the earliest recommendations were made by Kennedy (1955), who suggested that taking insulin usually poses few problems in the young diabetic and that children 8–10 years old or older can be trained to take over its administration completely. Subsequent work has not supported these early claims. Etzwiler (1962) asked 74 children attending diabetic camp to complete a questionnaire covering a range of information necesary for self-care. Although 75% of the 6- to 7-year-old children could interpret the results of urine tests adequately, only 50% of the older groups (16–17 years) could relate this information to their insulin needs. These data led Etzwiler to argue that the diabetic child should not be made responsible for self-care as young as Kennedy (1955) stated. Later work has continued to support this position.

Etzwiler and Sines (1962) extended the previous work by asking parents, teachers, camp counselors, and physicians of diabetic children to complete questionnaires about knowledge of diabetes. Etzwiler and Sines concluded that many parents as well as their children lacked the knowledge necessary for successful management. Of limited interest (since they are not broken down by age) are some data about who was responsible for various aspects of management of the disease. In the case of urine testing, it was reported that complete responsibility was taken by 88.7% of children, 45.8% of mothers, and 19.4% of fathers. For insulin injections the figures were 36.1% of children, 80.6% of mothers, and 26.4% of father. Collier and Etzwiler (1971) analyzed the type of errors most frequently made by diabetic children in answering the questionnaire described above. Most frequent errors apparently involved failure to recognize symptoms of acidosis, testing for acetone, knowledge of different varieties of insulin, and items to do with dietary control. In a similar analysis of common errors, Garner and Thompson (1974a) reported that lack of knowledge of genetics, diet calculation, and identification of symptoms relating to control were most common, especially for children between 9 and 13 years of age. More than half of the children described a diabetic diet as composed of "special foods" rather than a "well-balanced diet that the whole family can use." In addition, a high proportion of the children stated that diabetic care involved "rigidly following the rules for control, not engaging in unusual activities, and always asking the doctor before doing anything different" (Garner, & Thompson, 1974b, p. 246). Such an approach does not seem indicative of the type of self-responsibility for care that most pediatricians would hope for.

The type of information Etzwiler (1962) and Etzwiler and Sines (1962) asked of patients was of both a theoretical and practical nature. It is possible, however, for patients to manage their disease quite adequately, even without knowledge of theoretical aspects of the disease. For this reason, recent work has included assessment of children's skills at urine testing and insulin injections, instead of relying purely on factual knowledge. Thus, Garner, Thompson, and Partridge (1969) and Garner and Thompson (1974b) were interested in children's and parents' abilities to demonstrate without using food scales the servings of five different foods that represented a given weight. Gross errors in estimation were recorded. Further, there was no relationship between children's scores on a general information questionnaire with their ability to judge accurately appropriate-sized servings of food. Malone et al. (1976), compared children's own urine test results with technicians' results from the same samples. There was agreement between children's and technicians' results in only 41% of cases, and in 41% of the tests children underestimated the amount of sugar present. A very simple task was set children by Epstein et al. (1980). Children dropped a tablet into a urine–sugar solution and were to compare the resulting color with the appropriate color chart. Even given this very simplified component or urine testing skill, 53% of the judgments were erroneous.

Attempts to relate children's general knowledge about diabetes and their skills in management tasks have been reported by Johnson et al. (1982). One hundred and fifty-one diabetics, aged between 6 and 18 years, and 179 of their parents participated in the study. Three aspects of knowledge were investigated. The first was a multiple-choice questionnaire, covering children's knowledge about the cause of diabetes, the meaning of common terminology, and facts about treatment. This aspect of the study was similar to the approach described above (Etzwiler, 1962). A second questionnaire was described as "problem-solving." Situations were described that a diabetic might commonly encounter; examples are shown in the following list. Thirdly, "skill" was measured by observing children test a standard 7% sugar–urine sample and preparing an appropriate insulin injection.

*Examples of problem-solving questions used by Johnson et al. (1982)**

1) You are at a school football game and begin to feel dizzy, shaky and faint. What should you do?
    a) Leave the game right away and go straight home.
    b) Buy a coke and hot-dog and eat them.
    c) Lie down, until you feel better.
    d) I don't know.
2) You have the flu, with a high fever and don't feel like eating. You check your urine and it is 8% and large. You should:
    a) Hold your morning insulin because you're not eating as much.
    b) Add regular insulin to your usual morning dose and call your doctor.
    c) Do nothing different because everybody gets the flu.
    d) I don't know.
3) You are trying out for the swimming team and practice is mid-afternoon. Your urine tests are usually negative before lunch and in mid-afternoon. You should:
    a) Decrease your insulin the days you practice.
    b) Eat a particularly big lunch that day.
    c) Increase your insulin to give you more energy that day.
    d) I don't know. (p. 709)

On the skills test, older children were more accurate than younger, and girls of all ages were more accurate than same-aged boys. Eighty percent of the children made significant errors on urine testing, and 40% made errors on self-injection. Skills in both these areas were not

*Copyright American Academy of Pediatrics, 1982.

correlated with children's knowledge of diabetes assessed by questionnaire. Neither was there any correlation between the length of time children had been diabetic and their knowledge of the disease. Johnson et al. concluded that children's knowledge was insufficient to make daily management decisions. They further hypothesized that children should be taught specific aspects of management at certain ages. Children were thought to be most receptive to information about diet and insulin reaction at 6–8 years, to information about self-injection at 9 years, and to urine testing at 12 years. These ages are considerably older than those suggested by Kennedy (1955).

A similar approach was adopted by Harkavy et al. (1983). These investigators were concerned both with children's knowledge of diabetes and skill at management before attending summer camp and in how much the children benefited from the camp experience. The children were aged between 10 and 15 years and attended camp for 2 weeks. Much of the data replicated the earlier findings of Johnson et al. (1982), for example, the degree of knowledge was not very adequate, girls were more accurate in skills tests than boys, and duration of diabetes did not predict the child's scores. Of interest, though, was the fact that 12- to 15-year-old children showed significant improvements both in their degree of knowledge and diagnostic skills over the 2-week period. No significant changes were noted for the 10- to 12-year-olds. The results may be interpreted as further evidence that cognitive maturity is important in determining what children know and *are able to learn* about diabetes and its management.

Similarly Eiser, Patterson, and Town (in press) assessed children's knowledge of diabetes using questionnaires and attempted to relate this to parents' reports of children's actual responsibility for management. The questionnaire consisted of 21 multiple-choice items covering the following aspects of diabetic management: the effects of exercise on insulin requirements, urine testing, insulin reaction, theoretical questions about the cause of diabetes, and diet. The percentages of children by specific age groups who gave correct responses to these questions are shown in Table 6-2. While some aspects of knowledge appear to increase in a linear fashion (e.g., insulin reaction, theoretical knowledge), others are poorly understood by the youngest group but managed adequately by both older groups (e.g., diet).

Data regarding the extent to which the child was responsible for managing the disease were obtained from parents. Fifty-four percent of the sample were reported to be totally responsible for testing their own urine; 54.7% of children also tested their own blood if necessary. Seventy-six percent of children prepared their own injections. The children were divided into two groups; those who were completely responsible for testing their own urine and those who were not. Children who were responsible for this aspect of management also scored higher on the questions related to urine testing ($\chi^2 = 9.98$

Table 6-2. Diabetic Children's Knowledge of Diabetes and Treatment: Percentage of Correct Responses as a Function of Age and Content

Knowledge	6- to 10-year-olds (%)	11- to 13-year-olds (%)	14- to 17-year-olds (%)	Total (%)
Diet	37	78	88	70.20
Insulin	60	78	94	78.24
Urine testing	60	61	96	85.26
Insulin reaction	48	74	89	71.93
Illness	43	56	78	59.65
Exercise	83	94	94	91.23
Theoretical	50	78	82	71.93

Note. From "Knowledge of diabetes and implications for self-care" by C. Eiser, D. Patterson, and R. Town, in press, *Diabetic Medicine.*

$p < .05$). This was not true, however, when a similar analysis was conducted comparing children who were reported to manage their own diet and those who were not. There were no differences beween these two groups in the scores on knowledge about diet ($\chi^2 = 2.08$).

Most of these studies have looked at the child's knowledge of various aspects of diabetes, and attempted to infer from this an age appropriate for self-management by the majority. A study by Partridge, Garner, Thompson, and Cherry (1972) asked children directly about when they had assumed responsibility for insulin injections, urine tests, and diet. Children were also asked what they considered to be the "ideal" age to assume responsibility for these and other more general behaviors. Younger children reported that they were responsible for managing their own diabetes at an average age of 9.1 years, but they believed that such responsibility should not be accepted until an average age of 11.9 years. On the other hand, teenage diabetics reported that they were responsible for managing the disease at an average age of 12.6 years, and at the same time they considered this ideal. As shown in Table 6-3, diabetics did not differ from nondiabetics in the ages at which they were responsible for behaviors not related to their diabetes. These data are important, since it is often stated that sick children in general and diabetics in particular are less mature and more dependent on others. The study by Partridge et al. (1972) represents one of the few studies to test this assumption empirically and offers no support for the claim.

Beliefs About How Diabetes Affects the Body

The studies reviewed so far have all been concerned with assessing children's factual knowledge about diabetes and its management. Others have focused more on children's understanding of the signifi-

Table 6-3. Diabetic and Nondiabetic Adolescents' Statements About Responsibility for General Behavior

Responsibility	Mean Age in Years	
	Diabetics	Controls
Choosing clothes	12.2	12.5
Managing money	12.1	11.7
Arranging transport	13.2	13.7
Choosing friends	7.4	7.8
Choosing recreation	9.2	10.6
Choosing hair-style	11.3	11.7
Key to own home	12.8	12.1
Outside part-time job	13.1	13.2
Night hours	13.8	14.3
Deciding diet	10.8	11.5
Chores at home	10.2	10.4

Note. From "Attitudes of adolescents toward their diabetes" by J. W. Partridge, A. M. Garner, C. W. Thompson, and T. Cherry, 1972, *American Journal of Diseases of Children, 124.* Copyright 1972 by the American Medical Association. Reprinted by permission.

cance of diabetes for body functioning. In this respect a study by Kaufman and Hersher (1971) is frequently quoted. These authors claimed that despite repeated and extensive teaching, children held some very basic misconceptions about how diabetes affected their bodies. Five adolescents were asked to draw the inside of their bodies. Some of the children believed that part or all of their pancreas was missing, others that it was completely filled with sugar. There were also gross distortions in children's estimates of the size of their stomachs compared with normal children's. Diabetics were reported to believe that they had especially large stomachs, since they required so much more food than healthy children.

These apparently quaint data have serious implications. Successful communication between doctor and patient is dependent on a shared language, and is hampered in situations where the patient holds a set of beliefs unknown to the doctor (Pendleton & Hasler, 1983). The data of Kaufman and Hersher (1971) imply that difficulties in communicating with diabetic children may be due at least in part to misconceptions such as these. The extremely small sample size necessitates further investigation of this hypothesis, however.

Eiser, Patterson, and Tripp (1984a) attempted a more detailed investigation of diabetic children's knowledge and understanding of bodily processes. Children were given an outline drawing of the human body (male for boys and female for girls) and asked to draw what they thought they looked like inside. They were then asked to explain the function of the following organs: heart, brain, stomach, lungs, liver, kidney, pancreas, and intestine. Finally, the children were asked if they knew what diabetes was and how it was caused. The children were aged between 6 and 17 years, and their responses were compared with those of a healthy control child of similar age and sex and attending the same school. In this study there were relatively few differences between diabetics and controls in their knowledge of the body. Thus, although older children in both groups named more parts of the body than younger children, there were no differences between the diabetic and control groups (see Table 6-4). There were, however, some differences beween diabetics and controls in terms of which body parts were drawn. Diabetics were less likely than controls to draw a brain ($\chi^2 = 5.07$, $p < .05$) or a stomach ($\chi^2 = 8.08$, $p < .01$). Naturally enough, diabetics were more likely to draw a pancreas ($\chi^2 = 18.50$, $p < .001$).

Children's explanations of the function of different body parts were coded along the lines described by Gellert (1961) (see Chapter 2). There was only one significant difference beween diabetics and controls in their knowledge of the function of body parts. Diabetics were more likely to offer an adequate explanation of the function of the pancreas ($\chi^2 = 17.10$, $p < .01$). It was previously reported by Kaufman and Hersher (1971) that diabetic children believed they had larger stomachs than normal children, since they were required to eat so much more food. Comparison of the size of stomach drawn by the two groups did not support this hypothesis.

Finally, the beliefs of the children about the cause of diabetes were investigated. Diabetic children were more likely than healthy children to believe that the cause of the illness was unknown ($\chi^2 = 4.42$, $p < .05$) or the result of failure of the pancreas ($\chi^2 = 34.64$, $p < .001$). On the other hand, healthy children believed diabetes to be caused by "eating too much sugar" ($\chi^2 = 12.34$, $p < .001$).

Eiser, Patterson, and Tripp (1984a) concluded that there were few quantitative differences between diabetics and controls in their knowl-

Table 6-4. Mean Number of Body Parts Named by Diabetic Children and Healthy Controls as a Function of Age

Group	6- to 10-year-olds (Mean)	11- to 13-year-olds (Mean)	14- to 17-year-olds (Mean)
Diabetics	2.20	4.64	5.76
Controls	2.86	4.52	6.82

Note. From "Diabetes and developing knowledge of the body" by C. Eiser, D. Patterson, and J. H. Tripp, 1984a, *Archives of Diseases in Childhood, 59*. Reprinted by permission of the British Medical Association.

edge of the workings of the body. There was a suggestion in the data, however, of differences in their beliefs about the relative importance of various parts of the body. The diabetics were less likely to draw a brain, and yet it was clear from their explanations of the function of the brain that they were as aware of its importance as the healthy children. One 15-year-old diabetic later explained that what happened in her head was of less interest than what went on in her insides. Such statements indicate that some of the previous confusion in the literature about the body-image of the chronically sick may be due to a lack of precise definition of the terms involved. Future work needs to examine not only children's academic knowledge of their bodies but also the perceptions and attributions of the relative value of various body parts. This distinction was tentatively made by Shontz (1971), but there has been little attempt to apply it systematically to research.

Knowledge About Future Complications

However well-controlled diabetes is, the risk of serious complications developing in the future is very real, especially for those developing diabetes during childhood. Both Fallstrom (1974) and Galatzer et al. (1977) reported that "worries about future complications" was one of the "worst" things about diabetes according to sufferers. Gil, Frish, Amir, and Galatzer (1977) suggested in fact that children and parents may be more worried about long-term complications than is realistic. In this study parents and children were asked how likely they thought various complications of diabetes were, and how long since diagnosis before such complications might be expected. In most instances, parents rated the likelihood of complications as greater than that estimated by children. Gil et al. suggested that the lower estimates given by children might account to some degree for their lack of compliance to medical regimes. In the study by Eiser, Patterson, and Town (in press) parents were asked about their particular concerns both for the present and in the future. For the present, parents were worried about physical complications (4.3%), overweight (6.5%), cheating over food (4.4%), general control (34.7%), and "other" (15.3%). The percentage of parents who stated that they had no worries at all was 34.7%. In contrast, parental worries for the future were primarily in terms of physical complications (50.0%), pregnancy (10.9%), jobs (11.0%), control of food (10.8%), and general worries (8.7%). The number of parents with no worries was slightly less (12.9%).

Intellectual Development and Academic Achievements

As has been suggested, diabetes appears to be one of the more preferable chronic illnesses. Children with diabetes do not look different from others, and do not experience regular, very painful medical procedures. Neither are they required to consume vast quantities of drugs. In three separate studies, in fact, it has been reported that diabetic children do not describe themselves as different from others (Davis et al., 1965; Delbridge, 1975; Partridge et al., 1972). What sets them apart from others is their regular need for food, especially in relation to exercise, and of course, the daily urine sampling and insulin injections. For most children, life at school should be relatively free of problems. Urine tests and insulin injections are usually dealt with entirely at home, so that the main problem in school is reduced to one of eating enough to balance the child's needs.

Despite these arguments, some early writers felt that the diabetic child was unlikely to attain above-average intelligence levels. Teagarden (1939) for example, suggested that neurological and psychological functions may be impaired by diabetes and that insulin shock may produce neurological damage. Most early investigators, however, concluded that the intelligence of diabetic children did not differ significantly from the distribution among healthy children, (Brown & Thompson, 1940; Fischer & Dolger, 1946; McGavin, Schultz, Peden, & Bowen, 1940).

These general conclusions were also reached by Ack et al. (1961). In this latter study, 38 diabetic patients (aged between 3 years and 1 month and 18 years and 6 months) were compared with their siblings. Intelligence was measured using the Stanford-Binet Scales. Ack et al. do not report mean IQ scores, but rather they were interested in IQ differences between patient and sibling. Thirteen patients had been diagnosed before 5 years of age; the remaining 25 after 5 years of age. Patients diagnosed after 5 years of age had scores essentially the same as their siblings (average difference in IQ was +720 points). Patients diagnosed before 5 years had significantly poorer scores than their siblings (average difference in IQ was −10.15 points). Ack et al. hypothesized that biochemical changes in the brain resulting from diabetes are likely to be more damaging to the immature compared with the more mature brain.

This finding has not been pursued by later researchers. However, some degree of problems in school for diabetic children was noted by Fallstrom (1974). Problems were only significant among unstable diabetics, according to Koski (1969), and did not develop until higher rather than elementary school grades (Laron et al., 1972). In a study primarily concerned with identifying behavioral and psychiatric problems among diabetics, Gath, Smith, and Baum (1980) reported that twice as many diabetic children as controls had serious reading difficulties in school. Backwardness in reading was unrelated to hypoglycemic attacks, but children with poor clinical control were more likely to be poor readers than children with good control. (This result is presumably mediated by social conditions; inadequate social background being associated both with poor control of diabetes and also with low achievement in school.)

There are neither theoretical nor empirical grounds for supposing that diabetes affects a child's intelligence. There is, however, at least some evidence that the disease, or its associated treatment, does limit the child's potential. Such research as there is into the occupational status of diabetics support this view (Tattersall & Jackson, 1982).

Effects of Diabetes on the Family

Like all chronic illnesses, diabetes disrupts family life. It may be a relatively "desirable" condition, but for those who have to live with it, diabetes threatens the nature of family life. Parents must face the fact that their child has a potentially life-threatening condition and learn to cope with it. This means making adjustments to the family's diet, either by cooking specially for the sick child, or changing the whole family's diet in order that all family meals adhere to the same restrictions. Daily urine examinations and insulin injections must be fitted round other activities. At times when the child's control is poor, these tests have to be increased in frequency. In addition, increased anxieties about long-term effects become especially critical. It is easy for others to underestimate the anxiety generated for parents in balancing the complex demands of the child's diet, exercise and health.

Bruch (1948) identified three ways in which mothers appeared to cope following a diagnosis of diabetes in their child. These were defined as (1) tolerant and relaxed acceptance, (2) perfectionist overcontrol, (3) erratic or poor cooperation. Bruch further found that attitudes of tolerant acceptance were the least frequent. Most mothers were described as showing erratic or poor control. Where mothers adopted a policy of "perfectionist overcontrol," satisfactory regulation of the disease occurred, but the children were susceptible to behavior difficulties and poor schoolwork.

Swift, Seidman, and Stein (1967) compared family functioning for 50 diabetic children and 50 controls. Greater anxiety, hostility, and dysphoria were characteristic of the families of diabetics. Crain, Sussman, and Weil (1966) studied marital relations between parents of diabetic children and parents of "normals." Parents of diabetics scored more poorly on four measures of marital functioning. None of these studies, however, address the question of how diabetes affects a family, as distinct from any other chronic condition. Studies comparing diabetic families with those with a different threatening illness and with normal families are necessary to answer this question but have not yet been attempted.

There can be no doubt that psychosocial variables related to family functioning are important in determining the child's compliance with medical regimens. Schafer, Glasgow, McCaul, and Dreher (1983) measured adherence to medical regimens and metabolic control in 34 diabetic adolescents and related these data to measures of family functioning. These measures were both specifically related to diabetes, including a Diabetes Family Behavior Checklist (Schafer et al., 1983) and also of more general relevance (e.g., Moos Family Environment Scale (Moos & Moos, 1976).

Schafer et al. (1983) concluded that patients were not simply "good" or "poor" adherers to treatment, as much of the early literature suggests. Rather, it was more common for patients to conform well in some areas of their treatment (e.g., diet), while being much poorer in adherence to others (e.g., urine testing). They speculate further that different psychosocial variables might determine adherence to various aspects of disease management. An additional finding was that measures of family functioning specifically concerned with diabetes management were more predictive of adherence than general measures of family interaction (i.e., as measured by the scale in Moos & Moos, 1976). Finally, it was noted that these measures of psychosocial variables did not predict the child's degree of metabolic control. However, "control" is especially difficult during adolescence, the age of the children in this study. This is probably due to hormonal changes typical of adolescence and results in greater difficulty to maintain good control. It would be interesting to repeat the study with younger patients, in whom the relatively slower growth rate is more conducive to good control.

An important study by Garner and Thompson (1974a) observed mother, father, and diabetic child triads participating in a series of tasks. Interactions between the triads were rated on a number of variables including "comfort." Coping techniques used by the most "comfortable" families followed a traditional pattern. The child assumes low status compared with the parents and accepts it, sees himself or herself as like other siblings and the mother as more forceful than the child would like. It was notable that in comfortable families, both the child and parents were open about the child's diabetes. In this way, Garner and Thompson felt that any anxiety associated with the disease was mastered.

Few prospective studies of the impact of diabetes over time have been reported. Most researchers attempting comparisons between diabetic families and normals have not been clear as to how long the child has had diabetes. Clearly, family functioning is likely to be dependent on variables such as time since diagnosis of the disease. Koski (1969) provided some information about coping during the 1st year. Sixty children were divided into two groups on the basis of their diabetic control. Data were obtained from parent and child interviews, tests, observations, and teacher questionnaires. As documented elsewhere, families reacted first with a mixture of bewilderment, shock, and guilt, but reasonable patterns of adjustment were found within a few weeks. Mothers of children in good control were more expressive and emotional in their initial reactions, while mothers of children in poor control tended to be less expressive and denied any strong emotions. Children responded almost without exception with heightened anxiety during the time of initial medical procedures, but it is not clear exactly what aspect of the diagnosis and treatment contributed most to this anxiety.

It was parents' later coping behaviors that enabled Koski to make the distinction between the two groups. Parents' anxiety declined over time. Parents of those in good control tended to emphasize what was normal about the child's life, while at the same time adhering to the treatment regimens.

Koski and Kumento (1975) followed up these same families 5 years later. Nine cases originally found to be in poor control were then found to be in good control. A small number of cases changed from good to poor control, and a high incidence of family disruption was noted in these cases.

Preliminary data also of a longitudinal nature have been reported by Kovacs (1981). She is attempting to describe psychosocial reactions of the child and family during the first 5 years following a diagnosis of diabetes. Her findings indicate that mothers react more emotionally than fathers to the diagnosis, and approximately one third of mothers show clinically significant levels of depression. This acute adjustment period typically lasts around 6 months.

Minuchin et al. (1975) attempted to describe the relationship between family interaction and chronic illness. They suggested two ways in which psychological factors might influence control of diabetes. First, emotional disturbance might result in behavior problems, such as refusing to take insulin or diet properly, and this might have metabolic consequences. Alternatively, emotional disturbances might more directly have metabolic consequences. This was defined as "psycho-somatic" diabetes. In later work, they studied the effect of the family in producing this so-called psychosomatic diabetes.

Such families can be described in the following ways: (1) They show "enmeshment" to such an extent that individual identities and roles are unclear; (2) there is overprotectiveness to all family members; (3) there is rigidity in maintaining the "status quo"; and (4) there is a lack of conflict resolution. The sick child's role in avoiding family conflict is vital. When conflict does occur, there is accompanying emotional arousal—the "turn-on" phase. For the psychosomatic family, the "turn-off" phase is difficult, because the family attempts to avoid conflict with a consequent lack of conflict resolution.

Some empirical support for the model has been reported (Baker,

Minuchin, Milman, Leibman, & Todd, 1975; Minuchin et al., 1975). Some children with diabetes who were subject to a "stress" family interview showed an increase in arousal and free fatty acid production that did not turn off when the interview was finished. Although the model may adequately explain some children's reactions to family stress, it is not clear how frequently cases of psychosomatic diabetes occur. Of more importance, it is not known if such children have a heightened degree of anxiety regardless of the situation; in these cases the interaction in the family may simply be part of a wider problem with the child's functioning generally.

Some conflict between parent and child is likely to be due to differences in perceptions of the severity and implications for the future by the two groups. Ahlfield, Soler, and Marcus (1983) asked 50 diabetic teenagers and their parents to complete a questionnaire about daily life situations. Parents and children completed the questionnaire separately, and their answers were then compared. Agreement on the various items ranged from 30% to 86% (see Table 6-5). There was most disagreement for questions about scholastic performance, concentration, and social life. Male diabetics stated that the illness most affected their social lives, scholastic performance, and concentration, especially where the disease developed in children beween 9 and 12 years of age. Females believed that the illness affected their scholastic performance and concentration less than males. The parents of both male and female

Table 6-5. Agreement Between Diabetic Adolescents and Their Parents on Aspects of Daily Life

Aspects of Daily Life	Agreement (%)
Treatment by parents	86
Insulin injection	73
Child prepares meals	65
Relation with older siblings	64
Relation with younger siblings	55
Tell new friend about diabetes	51
Eat same foods	46
Eat at same times	42
Scholastic performance	45
Diabetes affects concentration	33
Diabetes affects social life	30

Note. From "Adolescent diabetes mellitus: Parent/child perspectives of the effect of the disease on family and social interactions" by J. E. Ahlfield, N. G. Soler, and S. D. Marcus, 1983, *Diabetes Care, 6*(4). Reproduced with permission from the American Diabetes Association, Inc.

diabetics perceived the disease to have a greater impact on their children's lives than did the children themselves.

Conclusions

Research on the psychosocial effects of diabetes has come a long way since the early focus on characterizing a "diabetic personality." There is an increasing recognition of the fact that patients should not be treated as passive recipients of medical care, but that the promotion of health and the prevention, detection, and treatment of disease are an individual responsibility (Strowig, 1982). The treatment of diabetes, more than that of any other disease, necessitates recognition of this attitude. Only by increasing knowledge of how the diabetic child and family perceive the etiology and limitations of the disease can we hope to understand the process of compliance with medical treatment and degree of metabolic control achieved by the child.

7

Asthma

Asthma attacks are frightening for child and parent alike. The sight of a child fighting for breath is likely to make parents fear for the child's life, and the constant threat of such an attack places a severe stress on the family. The problems are far from trivial; incidence of asthma tends to be high relative to other diseases. Simpson (1980) claims that 20% of children have one or more attacks of wheezing in the first 10 years of life. Peckham and Butler (1978) surveyed a representative sample of 11-year-old children. They reported that 3.5% had a history of asthma and a further 8.8% a history of "wheezing bronchitis." Both asthma and wheezing bronchitis appear to result from a single underlying defect, and much confusion arises because of the use of both terms (Williams & McNicol, 1969.) Other surveys (Morrison-Smith, Harding, & Cumming, 1971; Rhyne, 1974; Varonier, 1970; Williams & McNicol, 1969) are summarized by Kuzemko (1980), who concludes that the incidence of asthma is approximately 2%–3% for boys and 1%–2% for girls. Both the incidence of asthma and its severity are reported to be on the increase. Palm, Murcek, Roberts, Mansmann, and Fireman (1970) found both an increase in number of admissions and severity in a survey of hospital admissions in Pittsburgh.

Causes of the Disease and Treatment

Asthma has been defined as an illness that is manifest clinically by intermittent episodes of wheezing and dyspnea (shortness of breath) that is generally associated with a hyperresponsive state of the bronchi and may be antigen mediated. It is differentiated from other obstructive airway diseases by its unusual reversibility (Aaronson, 1972). Thus, "asthmatics are likely to respond with attacks of wheezing and shortness of breath because their bronchi respond more readily to stimuli (including allergens) than do normal bronchi. This wheezing and shortness of breath are generally only episodic, and the asthmatic child has symptom-free intervals" (Bronheim, 1978, p. 310).

Asthma can have an onset any time during childhood. Mortality rates vary from 1% (Barr & Logan, 1964; Ellis, 1975; Rackemann & Edwards, 1952) to 4% (Leveque et al., 1969). There is a commonly held belief that children "outgrow" asthma. Follow-up studies of children with asthma do not fully support this view (Kraepelien, 1964). Ellis (1975) studied asthma patients 20 years after the onset of symptoms, and reported that only 20% were completely symptom free. Blair (1977) studied 267 asthmatic children under 12 years of age and followed 244 of them after 20 years. At the end of the 20-year period, only 25% were symptom free. A further 25% had minimal symptoms, but the remaining 50% still suffered sufficiently seriously to warrant periodic hospital admissions or absences from work. Martin, Landau, and Phelan (1982) traced 336 childhood asthma patients when they were 21 years old. The authors concluded that two thirds of these subjects were still symptomatic. All of these studies suggest that children do not automatically outgrow asthma.

Etiology

Several factors, once identified as causes of asthma, are now believed to be triggering agents. *Allergens* of importance in childhood asthma include protein extracts of some forms. The most common allergens include inhalants, pollens, moulds, bacteria, and foods. Allergies to food most often include milk, eggs, and wheat products. Children can also be sensitive to house dust and animal dander. In cases where specific allergens can be identified, it is sensible to take steps to isolate the child from the allergens' influence. Where the allergen is the family pet, this may not be entirely easy to do.

Other variables, including a family history of allergic disease, stress, and infections, may trigger an asthma attack. Some authors have argued that the cause of asthma is in fact within the individual. Some evidence for physiological differences between individuals resulting in reactions to various stimuli in terms of bronchoconstriction have been reported. Agents that trigger attacks in asthmatics do not appear to affect nonasthmatics at all. Jones, Buston, and Wharton (1962) suggested instead that asthmatics have a chronic increase in bronchial lability, even when they are symptom free. In a subsequent report, Jones and Jones (1966) found that even adults who had been symptom free for at least 4 years had abnormally high bronchial lability. There is still no adequate explanation of the deficiency inherent in asthma.

Treatment

Although there is no definitive cure for asthma, many improvements have recently been made in treatment of these patients (Simpson, 1980). The purpose of treatment is to relax the bronchi. Home treatment involves medication by ingestion or inhalation. In addition, steps must be taken to reduce the incidence of attacks. For some children this may involve the exclusion of certain foods from the diet. For others who are allergic to dust and mould, thorough daily cleaning of the child's room or separation from pets and other animals may be necessary. For still others it may be desirable to reduce the potentially stressful nature of situations as far as possible.

Effects of Asthma on the Child

Personality Factors in Asthma

A psychological component in precipitating asthma attacks has been acknowledged since ancient times: Hypocrites reminded asthmatics that they should guard against their anger (Cohen, 1971). Later, Moses Maimonides (1135–1204), writing on asthma, suggested that "this disease has many aetiological aspects, and should be treated according to the various causes . . . it cannot be managed without a full knowledge of the patient's constitution as a whole . . . furthermore I have no magic cure to report" (cited in Cohen, 1971, p. 533). In the past, asthmatics have been described as overly dependent (Fine, 1963; Neuhaus, 1958), hostile and aggressive (Aaron, 1967; Alcock, 1960; Bacon, 1956), and emotionally unstable and neurotic (Fine, 1963; Miller & Baruch, 1967). Leigh and Marley (1956) and Dekker, Barendregt, and de Vries (1961) found that asthmatic children were more like nonasthmatic neurotics than normals.

Neuhaus (1958) compared 84 asthmatic children and their 25 siblings with 84 cardiac patients and their siblings. Both groups were then compared with a matched group of normal controls. Neuhaus concluded that asthmatic children were more neurotic, insecure, and dependent than normal children, but did not differ from their own siblings or children with cardiac disease. These data suggest that personality disorders must be the result rather than the cause of asthma, since they were also identified in a group of healthy siblings.

Graham et al. (1967) investigated the incidence of asthma and occurrence of associated behavior disorders. The sample consisted of all

9-, 10-, and 11-year-old children resident on the Isle of Wight in 1964. The incidence of psychiatric disorder according to both parents and teachers questionnaires was slightly higher for asthmatic compared with healthy children (10.1% and 10.7% for the asthmatics and 6.0% and 7.1% for the healthy children by parents and teachers, respectively). This difference did not reach statistical significance.

Williams and McNicol (1975) studied 400 asthmatics and 100 controls taken from a population of 23,000 school children. Assessments were made when the children were 7, 10, and 14 years old. In general, the group of asthmatics had fewer behavior disturbances than the control group. However, children with most severe asthma were more likely to show behavior disturbances than children with less severe illnesses. Such children were described as less socially mature, more demanding for material possessions or maternal attention, and more likely to exhibit unnecessary aggression.

Cernek, Hafner, Kos, and Cenlec (1977) compared 278 children suffering from asthma with 27 rheumatic and 19 diabetic patients. In addition, 105 normal healthy children were investigated. There were no differences between the four groups in IQ scores. Overall, however, asthmatic and diabetic patients were rated as more highly disturbed than rheumatic patients or normals.

While attempts to identify a cluster of personality traits specific to children with asthma have not been successful, more recent work has stressed how differences in personality might influence attitudes to the illness and consequent adjustment. Matus, Kinsman, and Jones (1978) investigated 72 patients with chronic childhood asthma. Patients were between 7 and 14 years old. All children were asked to complete a questionnaire containing 109 statements related to respiratory illness. The questionnaire was completed on two occasions, 1 week apart. Each statement was regarded as "conceptually representing an attitude such as denial of illness, stigma associated with asthma, level of realistic thinking about the illness, level of optimism, expectation about the patient's own role and that of others in its management, and orientation towards treatment personnel" (Matus et al., 1978, p. 612). Of the original 109 statements, 78 were selected as most discriminating and reliable. Subjects were asked to rate these on a 5-point scale (from strongly agree to strongly disagree). Cluster analysis of these items yielded seven factors: minimization of severity, passive observance of illness, bravado, expectation of staff rejection, moralistic authoritarianism, stigma, and external control. While some of these were unrelated to chronological age, three factors (minimization, expectation of staff rejection, and external control) were especially prevalent among the younger groups. Matus et al. (1978) concluded that attitudes toward asthma are quite stable throughout childhood. They suggest that during childhood the importance of magical beliefs declines and is replaced by greater bitterness. While older children associate action and involvement with exacerbation of the disease, younger children associate helplessness and passivity.

The approach taken by Matus et al. (1978) in investigating chronically sick children's attitudes to their illness is radically different from the open-ended interview techniques adopted by Bibace and Walsh (1981) and Brewster (1982). Yet the conclusions of all three studies are compatible. These data add further support to the argument that greater attention needs to be paid to developmental differences in children's perceptions and understanding of their illnesses.

Children's Knowledge About Asthma

A disturbing study by Martin, Landau, and Phelan (1982) points to a relatively poor level of knowledge about asthma among sufferers and an associated disregard for appropriate health-related behaviors. These authors studied 336 21-year-olds, who had begun wheezing before 7 years of age. Knowledge of asthma relating to the following four general areas were assessed:

1. Diseases associated with asthma
2. Factors likely to provoke attacks
3. Long-term effects of asthma
4. Drugs used in asthma management

Four grades of severity of the disease existing among the sample were identified: (1) subjects with a history of wheezing during childhood or adolescence but no incidences in the preceding 3 years before the age of 21 years; (2) subjects who had wheezed within 3 years but not within 3 months of the interview; (3) subjects who had wheezed within 3 months of the interview, but whose wheezing was neither frequent nor persistent; and (4) subjects with a current history of frequent (once a week or more) or persistent wheezing during the past year. Only subjects in this final category had an adequate knowledge of asthma. Martin, Landau, and Phelan (1982) concluded that there was also a high incidence of smoking among the sample. In that many childhood asthma patients are likely to continue to suffer from the disease into adulthood, there clearly is a need to increase understanding of the disease among this group.

Intellectual Development and Academic Achievements

There is undoubtedly a stereotype of the child with asthma having a preference for sedentary occupations, including reading, writing, card playing, and jig saw puzzles. Such observations led some early writers to claim that children with asthma were superior in intelligence and related academic achievements compared with healthy children. Evidence for such claims is not so clear-cut.

Piness, Miller, and Sullivan (1937) failed to show that children with asthma were intellectually superior. As mentioned, Graham et al. (1967) studied all children with asthma resident in the Isle of Wight. Compared with healthy controls, asthmatics tended to have slightly better school results. The asthmatic children had slightly higher scores on a test of nonverbal skill (almost at the 5% level) and were slightly better (but not significantly) on tests of reading and arithmetic. However, there was an overrepresentation of children from families of higher socioeconomic status and this may have contributed to the results. A study by Rawls, Rawls, and Harrison (1971) did little to improve understanding of the relationship between asthma and intelligence. In their study 199 boys and 172 girls with a history of allergic disease (as reported by their parents) were compared with a control group of 419 boys and 400 girls. Although teachers rated the allergic children as less intelligent, poor students, and low achievers, tests of reading, arithmetic, vocabulary, and block design failed to distinguish between the two groups.

Mitchell and Dawson (1973) studied the prevalence and educational and social characteristics of children with asthma resident in Aberdeen, Scotland. The authors identified 121 cases, giving a prevalence rate of 4.8%. They point, first of all, to the high school absence rate for asthmatic children: 88 children experienced interruptions in their schooling as a direct result of the asthma. Such a high absence rate needs to be considered when discussing the effects of asthma on a child's intelligence. Unlike the report of Graham et al. (1967), it was found that more children with asthma came from families of the lower compared with middle and upper socioeconomic status. Despite this, children with asthma had higher IQ scores; the mean score for children with asthma was 102 and for healthy children was 95. The measure of intelligence used, the Moray House Picture Intelligence Test, is probably not as widely accepted a measure of general intelligence or problem solving as, for example, the Wechsler scales. For this reason, the conclusions reached by Mitchell and Dawson (1973) that "our studies confirm the belief that children with asthma are more intelligent than their peers" (p. 470) needs further confirmation.

A comparable study was reported by Anderson, Bailey, Cooper, Palmer, and West (1983); they surveyed 9-year-olds in Croydon, England. Their data show that 11.1% of the cohort was reported by parents to have had an episode of wheezing within the previous year. School absence for children with a wheezing history was high: 58% had school absences because of wheezing, and in 12% of these cases, the absence amounted to more than 30 days. Compared with healthy controls, wheezy children had more atopic conditions, recurrent headaches, and abdominal pains. School absence was related to parental separation, nonmanual occupation of the mother, more than three children in the household, poor maternal mental health and lack of access to a car. While the child's illness had substantial repercussions for the mother and rest of the family, there were no apparent effects on the child's social activities, that is, wheezing children were as likely to belong to clubs or go swimming as healthy controls. In contrast, 42% of mothers felt that their own lives were disrupted by the child's illness. In addition, 29% of mothers reported that "special allowances" were made for the child because of his or her illness. Other authors reported that special arrangements had to be made concerning holidays, pets, and cleaning arrangements. All these effects were strongly associated with the number of days of school absence.

Teachers rated the child's social, psychological, and educational adjustment. There was no relationship between reading age and number of days absent from school. Only for children who missed at least 30 days schooling was there any effect, according to teacher's ratings, on social and emotional behavior. Anderson et al. (1983) concluded that asthmatic children who experienced a high level of school absence are at an educational disadvantage. They also point to the interaction between social and cultural factors and the child's health as reflected in school attendance.

Effects of Asthma on the Family

Probably more than with any other disease, the contribution of social factors to the course and severity of childhood asthma has always been emphasized. Current thinking about the interaction between social and physiological factors are summarized in Figure 7-1 taken from Mattson (1975). It can be seen that this model is essentially an extension of that proposed by Pless and Pinkerton (1975) to account for general effects of chronic illness, applied specifically to the case of asthma.

Early work suggested that asthma was associated with a disruptive mother–child bond (Abramson, 1954). The asthmatic child was hypothesized to be overly dependent on the mother, such that any threat of separation could initiate an attack. Wheezing was equated with the child's suppressed crying for the mother. Some writers (French, 1950; French & Alexander, 1941; Saul & Lyons, 1951; Weiss, 1950) argued that crying is a means to reestablish the dependent bond and asthma develops when the crying is no longer tolerable to the mother. Miller and Baruch (1948) for example, compared 63 allergic with 37 non-allergic children. In their study 98% of the mothers of allergic children and 64.8% of the mothers of nonallergic children were classified as "rejecting." Many other research reports (Epstein, 1963; Fine, 1963;

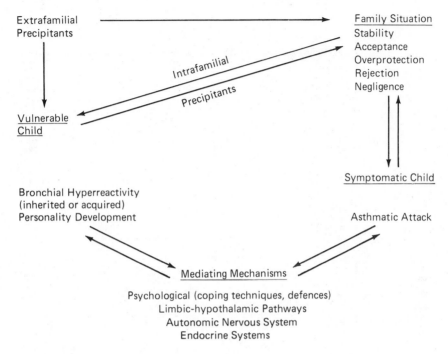

Figure 7-1. Interaction model of childhood asthma (Mattson, 1975). W.B. Saunders Co., 1975. Reprinted by permission.

Greenfield, 1958; Harris, Rapaport, Rynerson, & Samter, 1950; Little & Cohen, 1951; Long et al., 1958; Morris, 1959) and clinical case studies (Coolidge, 1956; Mitchell, Frost, & Marx, 1953) appeared to support the dependency theory.

Much of this early work, however, was methodologically unsound. Freeman, Feingold, Schlesinger, and Gorman (1964) made the following criticisms of the early literature: (1) Most work was based on groups of patients referred for psychiatric treatment. This deviant population should not be considered in any way as representative of the general population of asthma patients living with their parents and not referred for psychiatric treatment. (2) Medical diagnoses were often questionable, in some cases being based on self-report by psychotic patients. (3) There was often little attempt to ensure blindness of raters. (4) Most of the studies were post hoc, with no attempt to account for the fact that any disturbance in the mother–child relationship might be attributable to the course of the disease, rather than responsible for its onset.

Other studies, based on more acceptable empirical methods, have not found differences in the mother–child relationships in asthma (Cutter, 1955; Dubo et al., 1961; Fitzelle, 1959; McLean & Ching, 1973). Clearly, however, for a subgroup of children with asthma, the family

Table 7-1. The Schedule of Recent Experience (Coddington, 1972)

Experience	Preschool Score	Elementary Score	Junior High Score	Senior High Score
Beginning nursery school, first grade, or high school	42	46	45	42
Change to different school	33	46	52	56
Birth or adoption of a brother or sister	50	50	50	50
Brother or sister leaving home	39	36	33	37
Hospitalization of brother or sister	37	41	44	41
Death of brother or sister	59	68	71	68
Change of father's occupation requiring increased absence from home	36	45	42	38
Loss of job by a parent	23	38	48	46
Marital separation of parents	74	78	77	69
Divorce of parents	78	84	84	77
Hospitalization of parent (serious illness)	51	55	54	55
Death of a parent	89	91	94	36
Death of a grandparent	30	38	35	36
Marriage of parent to stepparent	62	65	63	63
Jail sentence of parent for 30 days or less	34	44	50	53
Jail sentence of parent for 1 year or more	67	67	76	75
Addition of third adult to family (e.g., grandparent)	39	41	34	34
Change in parents' financial status	21	29	40	45
Mother beginning to work	47	44	36	26
Decrease in number of arguments between parents	21	25	29	27

Increase in number of arguments between parents	44	51	48	46
Decrease in number of arguments with parents	22	27	29	26
Increase in number of arguments with parents	39	47	46	47
Discovery of being an adopted child	33	52	70	64
Acquiring a visible deformity	32	69	83	81
Having a visible congenital deformity	39	60	70	62
Hospitalization of yourself (child)	59	62	59	58
Change in acceptance by peers	38	51	68	67
Outstanding personal achievement	23	39	45	46
Death of a close friend (child's friend)	38	53	65	63
Failure of a year in school	38	53	65	63
Suspension from school		46	54	50
Pregnancy in unwed teenage sister		36	60	64
Becoming involved with drugs or alcohol		61	70	76
Becoming a full-fledged member of a church/synagogue		25	28	31
Not making an extracurricular activity you wanted to be involved in (i.e., athletic team, band)			49	55
Breaking up with a boyfriend or girlfriend			47	53
Beginning to date			55	51
Fathering an unwed pregnancy			76	77
Unwed pregnancy			95	92
Being accepted to a college of your choice				43
Getting married				101

Note: The scores are weighted for each life change, based on estimation of magnitude of life change. See text.
Note. From "The significance of life events as etiologic factors in the diseases of children" by R. D. Coddington, 1972, *Journal of Psychosomatic Research, 16.* Reprinted by permission of Pergamon Press, Inc.

environment is central in determining the course of the child's disease. As long ago as 1930, Peshkin (reported in Robinson, 1972) suggested that children with asthma might benefit from being separated from their families. While 10% of his patients remained asthmatic despite all efforts to manage them medically and remove allergens from their home environment, it was noted that they did become symptom free when hospitalized. At the same time, children were more likely to have asthma attacks on visiting days. Similar results were obtained during World War II (Bastiaans & Groen, 1955), when Dutch children with asthma were sent to boarding school in Switzerland. While the Dutch children appeared to improve in the mountain air, no improvement was seen among the local asthmatic children. After the war, Dutch children were sent to a local boarding school in Holland. Improvements in health were still noted, suggesting that what was critical was the removal of the child from the home environment, rather than any change in the "healthiness" of the environment. Further support for this argument is provided in the work of Long et al. (1958). They reported that hospitalized children with asthma remained symptom free when their rooms were sprayed with dust collected from the children's homes. More recent work also supports the view that removing the asthmatic child from the home environment can lead to improvements in the child's health. Unfortunately, it is also clear that the child's health is likely to deteriorate again on return home (Kapotes, 1977; Kellock, 1970; Peshkin, 1968; Sadler, 1975).

Boyce et al. (1977) investigated the role of stressful life events and family routines in triggering incidences of respiratory illness. They argued that stressful life events have been associated with patterns of streptococcal illness (Meyer & Haggerty, 1962) and occur more frequently in the year prior to general pediatric hospitalization (Heisel, Ream, & Raitz, 1973). In addition, they suggested that some aspects of the social environment might be *protective* against the impact of life change. Specifically, Boyce et al. (1977) suggested that a high degree of consistency or presence of strong family routines would protect the child against illness attacks.

Boyce et al. (1977) observed 58 children aged between 1 and 11 years for respiratory illness 5 days per week for 1 year. The children also underwent biweekly nasopharyngeal culture for pathogenic bacteria, mycoplasmas, and viruses. Each occurrence of illness (over the 1-year period) was rated by a nurse practitioner or pediatrician in terms of severity.

At the end of the year, the family of each child was interviewed, and a score for cumulative life change was calculated, based on the schedule of Recent Experience developed by Coddington (1972) for use with pediatric patients. A weighted score is assigned to a number of life changes (see Table 7-1; the score for each life change being based on its

Table 7-2. The Family Routine Inventory (Boyce et al., 1977)

Morning rituals
  Wake up at standard time
  Wake up by standard person
  Morning bath
  Dressing by standard person
  Breakfast each morning
Child's day schedule
  Nap each day
  Standard daily playtime activity
Meals
  Meals at standard time
  At least 1 meal eaten together
  Standard mealtime events at table
Homecoming
  Standard time for parental homecoming
  Greeting ritual for parent by child
  Greeting ritual for child by parent
Bedtime rituals
  Put to bed by standard person
  Put to bed at standard time
  Bath before bed each evening
  Sleeping arrangement constant
  "Good night" ritual (kiss, story reading etc.)
Chores
  Specific daily task (e.g., care, garbage, etc.)
Patterns of caretaking
  Standard weekly or daily care by person other than parent
Leisure
  Specific daily leisure event done with other family members
  Specific weekly leisure event done with other family members
  Specific daily or weekly leisure event done with persons outside family
Discipline
  Consistent, standard punishment for specified misbehavior
  Specific plan for parental sharing of discipline
Church
  Regular church attendance
  Home religious rituals
Visits to extended family
  Regular weekly or daily visits to extended family (grandparents, aunts, etc.)
Patterns of parents relationship
  Specific plan for parental sharing of child care or household tasks
  Scheduled, regular adult-centered event

Note. From "Influence of life events and family routines on childhood respiratory tract illness" by W. T. Boyce, et al., 1977, *Pediatrics, 60*(4). Copyright American Academy of Pediatrics, 1977.

estimated magnitude according to pediatricians, teachers, and mental health workers).

The Family Routine Inventory used in the study is shown in Table 7-2. One point was given for each routine regularly carried out by the family. An additional point was given if the routine appeared important to the family. The total score was thought to reflect the strength of family routines.

Boyce et al. (1977) made three conclusions. First, scores on the life change inventory were not related to the frequency of illness, but did predict how long a child remained ill. Second, severity of illness was related to an additive influence of life events and family routines. Greater life change together with a highly ritualized family may predispose an individual to greater illness severity. Third, neither the scores for life change events nor family routines were related to changes in microbiological parameters. In their conclusions, Boyce et al. emphasize the role of social factors in the etiology of respiratory disease, but acknowledge also that the exact processes involved are far from understood. The major strength of their study lies, perhaps, in the recognition of factors that may protect an individual against disease, as well as those that may increase susceptibility.

Conclusions

Asthma is one of the more common chronic conditions of childhood. Paradoxically, both the quantity and quality of psychological work on childhood asthma is inferior to that concerned with other chronic diseases of childhood. The early emphasis on inappropriate mother–child bonds in precipitating attacks has not been replaced by alternative research strategies. Many issues that have been considered worthy of study in relation to childhood diabetes have parallels in childhood asthma. There has been little interest in establishing how well informed the asthmatic child is about the condition, for example. Yet many children would be able to be personally responsible for controlling attacks caused by diet, exercise, house dust, or emotions. Few surveys have addressed the question of what the child with asthma understands about the condition, its cause, or its prognosis. The only exception (Martin et al., 1982) included a sample of 21-year-olds; the questions would be equally pertinent for a younger group. There are no data on the question of when the child with asthma should manage prophylactic aspects of the treatment that are comparable to the research literature organized around the age when diabetic children should manage their own disease.

Work with families of asthmatic children has also been less popular than work with families of other chronically sick groups. On the surface it could be argued that asthma imposes fewer demands on families and is generally less threatening than other illnesses. It is true that home treatment demands are generally less for asthma patients than for those with, for example, cystic fibrosis, renal disease, or diabetes. Hospital visits, too, are far less frequent. Nevertheless, as shown in the study by Anderson et al. (1983), families, and mothers in particular, can be seriously affected by the demands of the disease. The relatively high incidence of asthma should not lead to complacency about the psychological needs of this group.

In the final chapter on chronic diseases, we move from a relatively common disorder (asthma) to one of the least common (leukemia). Again it is apparent that much more work has been conducted regarding children with leukemia than regarding children with asthma.

8

Leukemia

The number of children affected by leukemia is small. Yet, excluding death by accident, cancer is the single most important cause of death in children, and acute leukemia is the most frequently occurring cancer.

Progress in treatment of leukemia has been dramatic. Untreated, the disease is invariably fatal within 6 months. Most medical centers offering specialized care for pediatric leukemic patients now quote survival periods of 5 years or more for 50% of patients (cf. Chessells, 1981; Li & Stone, 1976). These children "in remission" from the disease are to all appearances well. They must learn to live with a compromised existence, however, accepting both regular, routine hospital checkups and diagnostic procedures and the constant threat that the disease might return in a fatal form. Learning to cope with both the practical and emotional strains of the illness imposes immense pressure on the growing child, the family, and their interrelationships. Although media coverage of the advances made in treating leukemia have been extensive and created much public interest, considerably less has been reported nationally about the psychological implications of the disease.

Causes of the Disease and Treatment

There is no single known cause of leukemia, although viruses, radiation, and hereditary causes have been implicated in animal studies. There is a higher than expected incidence of leukemia among mongols and their families. Radiation is also known to be associated with increased incidence of leukemia, as occurred following the atomic bombings in Hiroshima and Nagasaki. However, many leading authorities now believe that leukemia is the result of a complex interaction of genetic, infective, radioactive, and other environmental factors (Allen & Cole, 1972; Willoughby, 1973).

The incidence of leukemia peaks among 4-year-old children (Willoughby, 1973). More boys than girls are affected. Iverson (1966), for example, reports that the incidence of leukemia in childhood is around 65 per 100,000 for boys and 46 per 100,000 for girls. Some 95% of cases of childhood leukemia are of the *acute lymphoblastic* type. A small number of children present with the *acute myelocytic* form. Treatment of this latter form has been far less successful than for acute lymphoblastic leukemia.

In simplest terms, leukemia is a failure of normal blood functioning by red blood cells. In healthy children, blood cells are formed in the bone marrow. *Red cells* carry oxygen to tissue, *platelets* prevent abnormal bleeding, and *white cells* defend against infection. In leukemia, abnormal white cells develop in the bone marrow and appear in blood and other tissue. The rapid increase of these abnormal cells inhibits production of normal cells and leads to the symptoms of the disease. On diagnosis, children are usually anemic (because of the decrease in normal red cells). They are often very lethargic and tired, pale, and may bruise easily. Children frequently present with bone pain.

Treatment

The usual method of treatment involves an intensive "induction" period of about 2 months followed by a period of "maintenance" for 2 years. Treatment beyond a 2-year period does not appear to extend the child's chances of survival (Nesbit, Sather, & Robinson, 1981; Medical Research Council, 1978). During the maintenance period, antileukemia drugs, particularly methotrexate, vincristine, and prednisolone, are used to destroy all identifiable leukemic cells in the child's body. However, since these drugs are not able to cross the blood–brain barrier in sufficient concentrations, some centers also treat the child by irradiation of the central nervous system (CNS). This reduces the risk of central nervous system relapse (Hustu & Aur, 1978; Medical Research Council, 1973). Other centers argue that such treatment is not necessary for successful outcome (cf., Freeman, Wang, & Sinks, 1977). In either case, after this initial period of induction the child can expect to be cared for on an outpatient basis, to return to school, and to lead as normal a life as possible. In part, this chapter is an attempt to determine the degree of success among children in achieving this aim.

Clinical Prognostic Features

There have been a number of attempts to define factors thought to influence the prognosis for the child with leukemia. Hardisty and Till

(1968), for example, reported an inverse correlation between survival and extent of disease on presentation. Children between 2 and 10 years of age generally have a better prognosis than very young or older children (George et al., 1973). Other prognostic indices are reviewed by Chessells (1981).

Effects of Leukemia on the Child

Personality Factors in Leukemia

Not surprisingly, children with leukemia often score higher on tests of anxiety than normal children. Waechter (1971) compared a group of children with fatal diseases (including leukemia and cystic fibrosis) with three other groups: (1) those with a nonfatal, chronic illness; (2) those with a brief illness; and (3) normal, healthy controls. Each child was shown eight pictures and asked to tell a story about each one. Children with a fatal illness were more likely than healthy children to tell stories involving overt death themes and to express concern about body mutilation or separation.

Spinetta, Rigler, and Karon (1973) compared 25 children with leukemia who were aged between 6 and 10 years with 25 children of comparable age suffering from chronic nonfatal diseases. Again, the children were assessed using a story-telling task and an anxiety questionnaire. Children with leukemia appeared more anxious than the children with nonfatal diseases about both hospital and home.

In a subsequent study, Spinetta, Rigler, and Karon (1974) investigated how such increases in anxiety and fear might affect the interpersonal relationships between children and adults. Children were given a doll to represent significant others (mother, doctor, nurse) and asked to place the dolls wherever they wished in a three-dimensional model of a hospital room. Patients with leukemia put the dolls at greater distance from the doll representing the self than those with nonfatal illnesses. Spinetta et al. (1974) argued that children cope with a fatal condition by progressively distancing themselves from others in anticipation of their own death. Spinetta and Maloney (1975) reported that even where leukemia patients were treated on an outpatient basis, rather than in hospital, they still became more anxious as the length of their illness increased. In contrast, children with chronic nonfatal diseases became less anxious during the course of their treatment.

Several studies point to an increase in incidence of behavior problems among children with leukemia. In one of the earliest of these investigations, Howarth (1972) reported that 40% of children with leukemia developed behavior problems. A figure of 31% was reported in a comparable study by Tiller, Ekert, and Rickards (1977). Maguire,

Comaroff, Ramsell, and Morris-Jones (1979) found that behavior problems were exhibited by 38% of children with leukemia compared with only 5% of those suffering from benign conditions.

Children with leukemia have also been reported to show behavior problems in school. Spinetta and Spinetta (1980) asked teachers of 42 children with leukemia to complete questionnaires about behavior in school, and these data were compared with those obtained from the teachers of 42 healthy children. Children with leukemia had more absences from school, were less able to keep up with the work, showed difficulty in concentration and learning, lacked energy, and were less willing to initiate activities or try new ones. They were also less likely to show physical affection or express their feelings, but more likely to cry, whine, and complain. Teachers rated 40% as exhibiting difficult behavior. A similar survey was conducted by Eiser (1980b). Again teachers reported that children with leukemia were behind with their schoolwork and had difficulty maintaining peer relationships.

Susman, Hollenbeck, Nannis, and Strope (1980) have taken a very different view in their own research. They argue that by focusing so much on the negative consequences of disease, investigators have neglected to note that much positive, resourceful behavior is also typical of the child with leukemia. Susman et al. point out that in all but the most exceptional circumstances, normal development does continue despite the experience of chronic illness. They argue that in most cases *development is not compromised to any significant degree*. Research should therefore attempt to describe the subtle ways in which chronic illness influences the process of development, rather than focus simply on measuring personality traits such as aggression or anxiety.

This approach is summarized in Table 8-1. In addition, Susman et al.

Table 8-1. Psychosocial Aspects of Cancer (from Susman et al., 1980)

Model 1	Model 2
Persons with cancer have psychological problems: Assess to detect pathology	Persons with cancer experience an atypical course of development: Assess to detect nature and frequency of problem
Diagnose the problems	Chart/professional mutual identification of goals/problems
Intervene to remediate pathology	Intervene to alter or maintain frequency of selected behaviors

Note. From "A developmental perspective on psychosocial aspects of childhood cancer" by E. J. Susman, A. R. Hollenbeck, E. D. Nannis, and B. E. Strope. In J. L. Schulman and M. J. Kupst (Eds.) *The child with cancer: Clinical approaches to psychosocial care—Research in psychosocial aspects.* 1980. Courtesy of Charles C Thomas, Publisher, Springfield, Illinois.

(1980) present some data based on these views. Children with metastatic solid tumors were observed for 15 minutes a day for 5 days a week. The author's findings led them to conclude that the manner in which chronically sick children may want to engage with others may be substantialy different from how others frequently do react to them. Thus, there is a tendency among adults to withdraw from a child in relapse, thinking the child to be weak, tired, and wanting to rest. Yet it may be especially at this time that the child needs to engage in social interaction, in order to alleviate fears of death. These data are preliminary, and the results no more than speculative. Yet this approach signifies a change in emphasis in dealing with cancer patients that can only be optimistic. As the authors themselves conclude, "It is our hope that with empirically generated findings based on actual behavior, the image of the child with cancer as a child who is depressed and anxious will be replaced with the image of a child who is hopeful, achievement-oriented, and enjoying interactions with others" (p. 142).

Children's Knowledge About Leukemia

In discussing leukemia with the pediatric patient, it is necessary to strike a balance between a not strictly honest, too optimistic view and one that is more pessimistic suggesting an inevitability of death, neither of which is totally justified. Many people believe that the cancer patient has a right to know about the illness, arguing that all but the very youngest children will work out for themselves that something is seriously wrong (Spinetta & Maloney, 1978). Despite the fact that most leading centers advocate answering the child's questions openly and honestly, the final decision rests with the parents. It is far from clear how many children understand the implications of their disease or at what level their understanding is. Of most importance, and essentially unresearched, is the issue of how, if at all, knowledge of the disease relates to the child's subsequent behavior.

In one of the few systematic studies, Morrissey (1964) studied 50 children with cancer including 42 children with leukemia. He found that only one third of the children were suspicious or aware of the disease, although most were highly anxious.

One study that looks somewhat indirectly at the child's understanding of the disease is by Mulhern, Crisco, and Camitta (1981). These authors were primarily concerned with communication patterns both within families and with physicians. Parents, physicians, and children rated probable survival times of the child. Physicians consistently gave less optimistic estimates of prognosis compared with mothers or fathers. Physicians underestimated mothers' and fathers' views, while both parents significantly overestimated physicians' views. Children's views of their own survival were higher than those of mothers or physicians, but did agree with their fathers' views. While both parents were aware of children's estimates of survival, physicians underestimated the children's views.

Mulhern et al. (1981) then conducted further analyses to determine what information was most relevant to the different groups in arriving at these estimates. For physicians, the child's age at diagnosis and white blood count (WBC) on remission accounted for 50.37% of the variance. Mothers' views were accounted for by the child's sex and duration of remission, that is, mothers were more optimistic about boys who had longer remissions. These factors accounted for 24.27% of the variance. For mothers, age at diagnosis, WBC, and Acute Lymphoblastic Leukemia (ALL) subtype were all noncontributory. Fathers' views were best predicted by the following variables; duration of remission, child's sex, age at diagnosis, and ALL subtype. The differences between the variables that contribute most to individual estimates of survival are probably very important; these data suggest that despite repeated explanations of the disease and its implications, parents consistently differ from physicians in their interpretations of these variables. While these data are important in indicating how parents arrive at their beliefs, they are less useful in understanding the child's awareness. One problem that always arises in connection with this question is that, because leukemia affects such young children, it is difficult to ask them directly about their knowledge or beliefs about the illness.

Similar discrepancies between parents and children in their knowledge and attitudes toward the disease were reported by Levenson, Copeland, Morrow, Pfefferbaum, and Silberberg (1983). Fifty-five cancer patients aged between 11 and 20 years were studied. A slightly modified questionnaire was administered to parents, who were also asked for information about the child's treatment. The questionnaire was divided into four sections, as follows:

1. Responses to tests and treatment
2. "Need-to-know" items
3. Responses evoked by information
4. Additional information

The actual interview schedule used is shown in the Appendix at the end of this chapter. Parents and children differed in their responses for three of these sections. These were responses to tests and treatments, need-to-know items and the helpfulness of additional information. Parents and children were in agreement on questions about responses evoked by information. Of the total 26 questions asked, 9 showed significant parent–child disagreement.

Issues of diagreement included the amount of test and treatment choices available to the patient, helpfulness to the patient of receiving additional information for self and family, and the importance of learning about a) the patient's self-help efforts and treatment concerns; b) the effects of alcohol, smoking, or drugs on the illness; and c) socio-personal concerns regarding ways to talk to friends and relatives about the illness. In each instance, the parents reported these issues to be more important than noted by their children. (Levenson et al., 1983, p. 38–39)

In conclusion, Levenson et al. (1983) note that the overall level of agreement between patient and parent was 48%, which may be contrasted with a figure of 58% agreement between healthy children and their parents in response to personal and impersonal health-related questions (Oliver, 1977). Levenson et al. argue that such discrepancies between cancer patients and their parents are especially damaging, since they are likely to hinder further the family's resouces for coping with the disease.

While both the studies by Mulhern et al. (1981) and that by Levenson et al. (1983) are important in describing differences between patients and parents in their perceptions of the disease, the study by Mulhern et al. (1981) is especially important in attempting to identify qualitative aspects of the information used in reaching these decisions. Mulhern et al. (1981) stress that the information used by parent and physicians to estimate the child's possible life expectancy differ. A similar analysis of the process underlying the patients belief system could be very neces-sary. In this respect it is likely that how the child learns of the diagnosis may be as important as what is learnt. While many researchers now argue that it is important to explain the diagnosis to the child patient, there have been few attempts to compare how children react when they are well informed compared with how they react when no information is given. One exception is a study by Slavin, O'Malley, Koocher, and Foster (1982).

Slavin et al. (1982) rated a group of long-term survivors of childhood cancer (n = 114) in terms of adjustment assessed by a psychiatrist and psy-chologist, independently. In addition, patients were interviewed about when they were informed they had cancer and whether the diagnosis was given by a parent, doctor, or by some other means (i.e, learned from friends). Patients were divided into the folloiwng three groups on the basis of how and when they learned the diagnosis:

1. *Patients who were informed early*. These case included diagnosis within the 1st year or by the age of 6 years for patients diagnosed in infancy.
2. *Patients who were informed late*. In these cases diagnoses were not given within the 1st year or before 6 years of age.
3. *Self-informed*. Patients were not informed by parents or physicians. They learned the diagnosis through friends, by reading hospital charts, or by a process of deduction following a media program about cancer.

The results showed that of 59 children diagnosed before the age of 6 years, 30 were informed early, 19 were informed late, and 10 were self-informed. Of 55 children diagnosed after the age of 6 years (excluding 2 whose adjustment was not assessed), 18 were informed early, 12 were informed late, and 13 were self-informed. Children who were informed early had better adjustment ratings than those who were informed late or self-informed.

As hypothesized by others (Binger et al., 1969; Vernick & Karon, 1965; Waechter, 1971) the important variable may not be information as such, but the degree of openness and candor within the family. Thus, the degree to which parents are prepared to discuss the diagnosis with the child may reflect broader, more flexible attitudes to communication within the family, which is what determines the adjustment shown by the child. More detailed studies of communication within families with a leukemia child would be necessary to answer this question. Nevertheless, the data provide some evidence for those who advocate that children with leukemia should be informed about the disease—evidence that is based on empirical, rather than intuitive grounds.

Preparation of the Child for Treatment

The treatment of leukemia involves the child in some intensely painful procedures. Of these, bone marrow aspirations (BMA) are probably the most traumatic and painful (Jay, Ozolins, Elliot, & Caldwell, 1983). Children's reactions to bone marrow aspirations have been systematically investigated by Katz, Kellerman, and Siegel (1980). Katz et al. used an observer rating scale of anxiety in which observer ratings of 25 categories of behavior were recorded. It was reported that anxiety was inversely related to age and that younger children showed a greater variety of both verbal and physical expressions of anxiety over a longer time. In contrast, older children exhibited fewer signs of overt anxiety. Females showed more anxiety than males. It might be hoped that children would "habituate" or show less anxiety to the procedures over time, but this was not found to be the case.

A study by Jay et al. (1983) extended this previous work, by attempting to describe characteristics of patients showing most stress. These authors studied 42 pediatric cancer patients undergoing bone marrow aspirations. Consistent with the findings of Katz et al. (1980), it was reported that the younger children showed greater stress than older children. In fact, children under 7 years of age showed distress levels five times greater than shown by those over 7 years of age. These data are interpreted as indicative of cognitive maturity enabling children of 7 years or more to have a more realistic understanding of medical procedures, which functions to reduce anxiety. Although there were no differences between boys and girls in their levels of stress, it was found that higher levels of parental anxiety were directly related to higher levels of behavioral stress in the child. As pointed out by the authors, however, it is not clear which is cause and which effect—perhaps children who show extreme stress create more anxious parents. Jay et al. (1983) found that children habituated to the procedures, but unlike Katz et al., these authors suggested that habituation may take as long as 2 years, especially for children below 7 years of age. The tendency of younger children to show their anxiety by overt and noisy behaviors should not lead to neglect of the older, less demanding patients. Jay et al. concluded that children over 7 years reveal their stress through self-report measures rather than overt screaming. Despite this, the need for therapeutic intervention should not be neglected. Jay, Elliot, Ozolins, and Olson (in press) have detailed a number of behavior therapy techniques aimed at reducing stress in these patients. The methods adopted include filmed modeling, reinforcement, breathing exercises, imagery, and behavioral rehearsal. They report considerable success in the use of these techniques.

Intellectual Development and Academic Achievements

As the numbers of children successfully treated for leukemia increased, there developed a concern for the "quality of life" of the survivors. A central question was whether children suffered any deleterious consequences of prophylactic CNS treatment by irradiation. Early studies were reviewed by Furchgott (1963) and included not only research concerned with leukemia children, but also studies of children treated by cranial irradiation for tinea capitis and brain tumors, as well as the effects of whole body exposure following nuclear bomb fallout. Two opposing views on the vulnerability of the brain to irradiation can be identified. On the one hand, it has been argued that only developing and dividing cells are vulnerable, and since permanent cells are formed in the brain relatively early, little damage is likely (Furchgott, 1963). This view is based on some empirical evidence that shows that functioning is not inhibited following exposure to irradiation. An alternative viewpoint is that much brain development continues at least until 5 years of age (Dobbing, 1968). Additional evidence suggests that patients who receive cranial irradiation can show brain necrosis and other signs of encephalopathy (Oliff, Bercu, & Dichiro, 1979; Peylan-Ramu, Poplack, & Pizzo, 1978; Shalet, Beardwell, Twomey, Jones, & Pearson, 1977). Others have argued that irradiation does affect development, though indirectly, and is brought about by damage to the cerebrovascular system, which results in interference to the blood supply to the brain (Allen, 1978; Price & Jamieson, 1975).

The ideal experimental design to investigate this question might involve a comparison of a group of children randomly assigned to treatment for leukemia by CNS irradiation and chemotherapy with a group randomly assigned to be treated by chemotherapy alone. It would further be desirable to have reliable estimates of the children's intellectual functioning and academic achievements prior to the treatment and, in addition, to assess the changes in intelligence quotients throughout the course of the disease. The prospective component is especially important, since the mechanisms whereby radiation might induce changes in the structure or function of the CNS are unknown. Suggestions that radiation interacts with intrathecal methotrexate to reduce the permeability of the blood–brain barrier (Price & Jamieson, 1975) point to the fact that changes in intellectual functioning might be expected over a period of time rather than immediately following treatment.

In practice, it has not been considered ethical to conduct such a randomized trial. Since CNS irradiation has generally been considered vital in extending the life expectancy of the child with leukemia, it was also considered unethical to withhold this treatment from some children, simply to satisfy experimental rigor. Researchers have therefore been forced to adopt alternative strategies. Some have favored comparing pediatric leukemia patients undergoing CNS irradiation with children suffering from solid tumors. The choice of this latter group is usually justified on the grounds that the children suffer a similar disease in terms of its potential threat to life; they are treated by body irradiation and chemotherapy (and often surgery). The vital comparison however, is between a group treated by CNS irradiation and a group treated by body irradiation; any differences in intelligence between these groups can, with reasonable certainty, be attributed to these procedures. Researchers have also managed to trace small numbers of children who for various reasons were treated for leukemia without CNS irradiation. More recently, some centers have opted to treat children by drugs alone, arguing that their success is comparable to that of treatment by radiation alone (Green, Freeman, & Sather, 1980). Both these situations have enabled some assessments to be made of children suffering from leukemia treated with and without CNS irradiation (Moss, Nannis, & Poplack, 1981).

An alternative strategy involves comparison of children who have leukemia with healthy siblings. The argument here is that, since patients and siblings share the same genetic and environmental background, they should have comparable intelligence levels. Differences between the two groups in favor of the healthy siblings could therefore be interpreted as evidence of the adverse effects of the disease or treatment on intellect.

In addition to this choice of comparison groups, researchers can opt to study the effects of irradiation either by a single assessment of children who have undergone treatment for several years, or by continuous assessment of children throughout treatment and, if possible, in long-term remission. The first method is of course considerably easier to set up and has consequently proved the more popular. Some prospective studies have appeared in the literature, but unfortunately the maximum follow-up period is usually only 12 or 18 months after diagnosis.

Retrospective Studies

Some of the earliest investigations concluded that CNS irradiation did not affect the child's intellectual development (Soni, Marten, Pitner, Duenas, & Powazek, 1975). They investigated two groups of children: (1) 14 children treated by CNS irradiation for ALL compared with 19 children with solid tumors treated by irradiation to other sites and (2) 5 children treated by CNS irradiation for ALL compared with 9 children treated for ALL but not by irradiation. Those treated by CNS irradiation did not appear to deteriorate intellectually compared with the other children, from which Soni et al. concluded that the treatment was relatively safe. Several criticisms can be directed at Soni's work, however. The sample size was very small. The children with solid tumors were not a matched group with the leukemia children. In fact, the mean age of the solid tumor group was 10 years and for the leukemic group, 5 years. Differences in outcome may be due to the greater maturity of the solid tumor group. Finally, with repeated testing, Soni noted that the solid tumor group showed an improvement in scores, while the leukemia children remained at the same level, which might indicate a lack of ability to benefit from learning situations among those treated by CNS irradiation. Nevertheless, two other reports suggested that leukemia or its treatment did not adversely affect children. Verzosa, Aur, Simon, Hustu, & Pinkel (1976) concluded that 5 years after treatment patients showed no untoward effects in educational, neurological, or behavioral status. Obetz, Smithson, and Groover (1979) found no differences in functioning between leukemia patients, which might be attributed to differences in treatment regimens. Unfortunately, later work has not been consistent with these early findings. (Eiser, 1978, 1980a; Eiser & Lansdown, 1977; Jannoun, 1983; Moss, Nannis, & Poplack, 1981; Stehbens, Ford, Kisker, Clarke, & Strayer, 1981; Twaddle, Britton, Craft, Noble, & Kernahan, 1983).

Eiser and Lansdown (1977) assessed 15 children with ALL and compared them with normal healthy children matched for age, sex, and socioeconomic status. The mean score for children beginning treatment after 6 years of age did not differ significantly from the mean score obtained by the controls. Children under 5 years of age on diagnosis scored significantly lower in terms of the General Cognitive Index of the McCarthy Scales (McCarthy, 1970), and also on the Quantitative, Memory, and Motor Scales. There were no differences between the groups on the scales measuring vocabulary and perceptual tasks, nor in reading age. Eiser and Lansdown suggested that the treatment used to control leukemia might be too aggressive for the under 5-year-olds.

In a follow-up study, Eiser (1978) tried to separate the effects of CNS irradiation from the effects of the illness. The study identified a small group of patients ($n = 7$) who had survived, having been treated by drugs alone with no CNS irradiation. These patients were compared with a group who had undergone the then routine treatment of chemotherapy and CNS irradiation. Inevitably, the groups differed in terms of their length of survival (mean time without treatment for the nonirradiated group was 33 months; for the irradiated group, 6 months). The mean full-scale IQ score on the Wechsler Intelligence Scale for Children (WISC) (Wechsler, 1974) for the nonirradiated group (102.4) was significantly higher than for the irradiated group (mean = 88.6), indicating that children with leukemia have lower IQ scores than might be expected from population means. The data suggest that both the age of the child and the timing of radiation treatment are critical determinants of subsequent intellectual development.

Subsequently, Eiser (1980a) assessed three groups of children. The first group consisted of 40 children who had been treated for leukemia; the second, 16 who had been treated for solid tumors; and the third, normal healthy children attending local schools. The healthy children were matched with sick children for age, sex, and socioeconomic status, and whether they came from a one- or two-parent family. The main measures of assessment used were the WISC and the reading ages. Scores on the WISC were converted to standard forms and then grouped according to the three factors identified by Kaufman (1975): verbal comprehension, perceptual organization, and freedom of distractability.

The children with solid tumors had scores on all these factors comparable with their controls, suggesting that despite the aggressive medical treatment and life-threatening nature of their condition, there were no measurable effects on intellect following recovery. The situation was very different for the children with leukemia, who scored consistently and significantly below their controls. In addition, separate correlations were conducted between the sick child's scores on the different tests with age of diagnosis. These correlations were significant for the groups of leukemia children, suggesting that scores on the IQ test decreased the younger the age of the child on diagnosis. There were no such correlations among the children treated for solid tumors. The data from this study suggest that normal intellectual development is possible even where children suffer from a life-threatening cancer. However, some aspect of the treatment appears to be implicated in the poorer performance of children with leukemia compared with those with other life-threatening cancers.

Stehbens, Ford, Kisker, Clarke, and Strayer (1981) assessed the intelligence of 38 newly diagnosed cancer patients with 29 patients with hemophilia. Their major finding was that the difference between scores on the verbal (VIQ) and performance (PIQ) scales of the Wechsler Intelligence Scale for Children—Revised (WISC-R) were greater for the cancer compared with the hemophilia patients. According to Wechsler (1974), a V–PIQ discrepancy of 15 points or more is significant at the .01 level. Stehbens et al. reported that 39% of the cancer sample showed a difference score of this degree, compared with 14% of the hemophilia sample. (This figure of 14% was reported by Kaufman [1976] to occur in the general population of 6- to 16-year-old children). Stehbens et al. also noted that increases of prednisone and vincristine correlated significantly with more negative V–PIQ discrepancies.

Kellerman, Moss, and Siegel (1982) reported an attempt to replicate these data. Among 45 newly diagnosed leukemia patients, Kellerman et al. reported that V–PIQ discrepancies were not different from those that would be expected for a normal sample. The authors point to several anomalies and methodological inadequacies in the original data presented by Stehbens et al. (1981). Perhaps the most pertinent were that (1) patients with a variety of cancers and not just leukemia had been included in the sample; (2) some patients were assessed after CNS irradiation had begun; (3) patients with chronological ages in the extreme range (6 and 17 years) were included; (4) only eight, rather than the usual 10 subtests had been used, and the data were prorated.

Subsequently, both Stehbens (1983) and Kellerman (1983) have made further criticisms of each other's work. It is unfortunate that this preoccupation with criticizing methodological aspects of each other's work has clouded the most important issue. Namely, even if it could be satisfactorily demonstrated that children newly diagnosed with leukemia showed deviant patterns of response on the WISC, several questions would remain to be answered concerning how these differences could have arisen. Although previous workers have not directly concerned themselves with such questions, there is a suggestion that patients who have received treatment for longer periods show lower performance rather than lower verbal scale IQ scores. What processes can be postulated to account for this apparent reversal in qualitative aspects of ability? Why should verbal scores be more affected by drugs than are performance scores? Stehbens et al. (1981) argued that depression or anxiety among these patients might account for the results, but no previous work satisfactorily suggests that either of these variables are associated with lowered verbal scores. Many newly diagnosed leukemia patients tend to be withdrawn and reticent in speaking to yet more adult strangers, and it is possible that the low verbal scores observed by Stehbens et al. are purely temporary and attributable to the child's confusion about what is going on. The possibility does of course remain that deviant IQ patterns are a result of therapy. Even so, the status of a Verbal–Performance IQ discrepancy score as an indicator of brain dysfunction has never been conclusive, partly because of the relatively high incidence of such discrepancies in the general population (Rutter, Graham, & Yule, 1970). Neither has there been any investigation of the implications of the discrepancy for education or remedial teaching. Until such implications are established, it seems premature to focus purely on the incidence of such a discrepancy.

Moss et al. (1981) compared 24 children with ALL with their healthy siblings. A significant difference in IQ scores between the groups, in favor of the siblings (112.5 vs. 98.6) was found. There was a marginally significant trend for the differences in scores between patients and siblings to be greater for children diagnosed at younger ages. In addition, Moss et al. compared a group of 13 patients with ALL, but who had not been treated by CNS irradiation, with their siblings. There were no IQ differences between these groups (mean IQ for ALL children = 102.8; for siblings = 98.7).

A similar experimental design was adopted by Twaddle, Britton, Craft, Noble, & Kernahan (1983). These authors assessed 23 children with leukemia (ALL) treated by CNS irradiation with their healthy siblings and 19 children treated for solid tumors and their healthy siblings. All the children were assessed using items from the British Ability Scales (BAS) (Elliot, Murray, & Pearson, 1978). The scores of siblings were used to estimate patients' IQ scores before treatment, according to the method described by McNemar (1962). This estimate of premorbid IQ was subtracted from each patient's score after treatment to give a change score. The study concluded that there was a "significant difference between the estimate before treatment and IQ scores after treatment in the ALL but not the ST group" (Twaddle et al., 1983, p. 951). The authors further argued that CNS irradiation was the major difference between the groups and therefore must be considered the primary cause. It was also found that the size of the change scores correlated with age, suggesting that greater damage to the CNS followed irradiation with younger rather than older patients.

Finally, Jannoun (1983) conducted the most extensive investigation to date. She traced 129 ALL patients and compared their performance with 67 healthy siblings by means of the British Ability Scales and WISC-R (Wechsler, 1974). The patients were divided into three groups as a function of their age at diagnosis. The youngest group had been diagnosed when less than 3 years old, a second group had been diagnosed between the ages of 3 and 6 years, and a third group had been diagnosed when over the age of 7 years. On the WISC-R the IQ scores for the two older groups were significantly higher than for the youngest group. This difference approached but did not reach significance when using the BAS. Where possible, patients' scores were also compared with those of healthy siblings. The mean scores for patients was significantly lower than that for siblings (101.3 and 111.8, respectively, $p < .001$). When this analysis was repeated separately for each age-group, it was found that the difference remained significant for the two younger groups but not for the oldest age-group.

Although many of the studies reviewed in this section may be criticized for inadequate sample size or poor selection of controls, the results are impressive in their consistency. Children treated between 2 and 3 years of age by CNS irradiation for leukemia subsequently have lower IQ scores than would be expected. In fact, there is now a move to delay CNS irradiation and treat very young children by chemotherapy alone (Chessells, 1981). A summary of these retrospective studies is shown in Table 8-2.

Prospective Studies

An alternative research strategy has been to assess children soon after diagnosis and again at intervals throughout treatment. It is assumed that this first assessment may be taken as a rough indication of the child's IQ prior to treatment and that any loss in IQ during the course of the illness is indicative of adverse effects of the treatement. Meadows et al. (1981) studied 31 children soon after diagnosis. Of these, 18 were retested between 12 and 34 months later. Scores on standard IQ tests and a neuropsychological test battery were compared with (1) six children with ALL who had received similar chemotherapy but no CNS irradiation and (2) six children with Wilms' tumors. (Again, the children with tumors had received similar chemotherapy but not CNS irradiation.)

Eleven of the 18 children with ALL showed a drop of 10 or more IQ points between the first and final testing session. Children aged between 2 and 5 years on diagnosis showed greater declines than those diagnosed when aged over 6 years. Wilms' tumor patients showed no significant change between testings. In fact, the median score increased from 102 to 114. It is undeniably difficult to assess intelligence in preschool children, and some might argue that the greater decrements observed in the very young children could be attributable to some artifact of the testing situation. On the other hand, it must be noted that the prospective data reported by Meadows et al. (1981) are consistent with the retrospective data reported in the previous section.

Tamaroff et al. (1982) studied 41 children with ALL treated by chemotherapy and no CNS irradiation. These children were compared with 33 receiving similar treatment for embryonal rhabdomysarcoma. One year after diagnosis there were no measurable differences in IQ

Table 8-2. Summary of Research on Effects of CNS Irradiation on Children's Intelligence Test Scores

Study	Leukemia Patients (n)	Comparison Group	IQ Test	Results
Soni et al., 1975	14	19 solid tumors	Stanford-Binet WISC	No effect
Eiser & Lansdown, 1977	15	15 healthy peers	McCarthy WISC	<5 years IQ of leukemia: 95.0 IQ of healthy: 114.6 $p < .02$ >5 years IQ of leukemia: 113 IQ of healthy: 119 (n.s.)
Eiser, 1980a	40	16 solid tumors 40 healthy peers	WISC-R	IQ of leukemia: 93.8 IQ of healthy: 105.8 $p < .001$ IQ of solid tumors: 101.4 IQ of healthy: 106.5 (n.s.)
Moss, Nannis, & Poplack, 1981	24	24 healthy siblings		IQ of leukemia: 98.6 IQ of siblings: 112.5 $p < .001$
Twaddle et al., 1983	23	19 solid tumors 23 healthy siblings	BAS	(data not presented in this form)
Jannoun, 1983	129	67 healthy siblings	BAS WISC-R	IQ of leukemia: 101.3 IQ of siblings: 111.8 $p < .001$

Note. CNS is central nervous system; WISC is Wechsler Intelligence Scale for Children; BAS is British Ability Scales; WISC-R is Wechsler Intelligence Scale for Children—Revised.

scores between the groups. Twelve of the youngest ALL patients were followed for 5 years from diagnosis, and still no decrement in IQ was found. These authors argue therefore that treatment for ALL is possible and desirable without CNS irradiation.

Stehbens, Kisker, and Wilson (1983) compared the intelligence, achievement, and behavior of children treated for leukemia with those treated for solid tumors at diagnosis and 1 year later. Although there were no changes in behavior ratings over the 1-year period for either group, it was found that children diagnosed with leukemia before 8 years of age showed declines in word recognition, performance IQ, and full-scale IQ. Both groups of patients aged 8 years or more on diagnosis showed no decreases in ability. The authors concluded that CNS prophylactic treatment used for leukemia patients is potentially aversive, at least for some children, and that any investigations need to take account of age in considering the child's prognosis.

The data of Stehbens et al. (1983) indicate that children with leukemia are at greater risk in terms of intellectual development than children treated for other cancers and that this risk is particularly great for very young children. While cross-sectional research suggests that these differences are apparent some years after diagnosis and treatment, the prospective study by Stehbens et al. shows that some declines are already apparent within the 1st year of diagnosis.

Effects of Leukemia on the Family

It would be naive to assume that the diagnosis of leukemia in a child might have anything but a traumatic effect. Certainly much psychological research supports this view. Binger et al. (1969) studied 20 families of children with leukemia and reported a high incidence of problems including family disturbance, difficulties with siblings, depression, and divorce. Kaplan, Smith, Grobstein, and Fischman (1973) found that 87% of their sample of families failed to cope well with the consequences of the disease. These people consistently denied the reality of the illness, were hostile to staff, did not inform the child, and did not communicate well with each other. Kaplan, Grobstein, and Smith (1976) found that only 21% of families remained together throughout the child's illness— a very depressing statistic. Peck (1979) investigated 24 families in which a child suffered from leukemia or Wilms' tumor. Parents were interviewed 4 years after diagnosis when all the children were well and in remission. Despite this, Peck reported that one third of parents were still extremely anxious, particularly about the possibility of a recurrence. Similar conclusions were reached by Tiller, Ekert, and Rickards (1977), working in Australia. They interviewed families 12 to 23 months after diagnosis of leukemia in the child, and found that 30% of mothers suffered a severe or moderately severe form of depression. Maguire et al. (1979) conducted a prospective study of the parents of 60 children treated for leukemia and followed them for the first 12–18 months after diagnosis. Parents were assessed using the Present State Examination (Wing, Cooper, and Sartorius, 1974) and the Standardised Social Interview (Clare & Cairns, 1978) and then were compared with a control group of parents whose children had been treated for benign disease. Maguire et al. (1979) found a relatively high incidence of problems for the families of the leukemia patients both in the period immediately following diagnosis and at follow-up.

In the period after diagnosis of the leukemia, 30% of the mothers were found to be suffering from an anxiety state. They felt on edge, were unable to relax, had difficulty getting to sleep, and found that they couldn't stop thinking about their child's illness. This compared with an incidence of 5% among mothers of children with benign disease. Over a third of the mothers of children with leukemia and 9% of mothers of children with benign disease also suffered from symptoms of depression. Twelve to eighteen months later a quarter of the mothers were suffering from an anxiety state or depressive illness compared with 8% of mothers of the control children. Maguire et al. (1979) concluded that a substantial proportion of mothers of children with leukemia develop psychiatric problems. Most of the problems could be described as mild or moderate in severity, but they tended to continue at least for the first 18 months following diagnosis.

In sharp contrast to these reports, there is a growing body of research that points to the immense resilience and extraordinary strength and coping abilities of families involved. Bozeman, Orbach, and Sutherland (1955) reported that especially during periods of remission parents were able to suspend thoughts about the loss of the child and function relatively normally. Four months after diagnosis mothers were found to be less worried and more hopeful than during the period surrounding diagnosis (Natterson & Knudson, 1960). Similar observations were made by Chodoff, Friedman, & Hamburg (1964) and Hamburg (1974). Using standardized tests of personality, Powazek et al. (1980) found that mother's distress lessened during the first 6 months of treatment. Nevertheless, and perhaps not surprisingly, anxiety, neuroticism, and neurotic maladjustment remained high. The longer the remission, the more likely families were to move toward a state of healthy denial or affirmation of life (Beisser, 1979; Friedman, Chodoff, Mason, & Hamburg, 1963; Futterman & Hoffman, 1973; Obetz, Swenson, McCarthy, Gilchrist, & Burger, 1980; Schulman, 1976).

It is difficult to reconcile such extreme points of view. Undoubtedly, treatment centers themselves differ in the way families are handled, and these results may in large part reflect differences in quality of care and psychosocial support. Also, it is of some doubt now how relevant very early studies are to the experience of patients today. Twenty years ago, it was not uncommon for patients to receive drug therapy for 5 years or more, a situation that would not now arise. Such extended periods of treatment are no longer thought advisable. A third source of these inconsistencies may be found in the research methodologies employed. Many reports were based on retrospective interviews conducted after the child's death, when parental perception may be significantly distorted (e.g., Binger et al., 1969; Lewis, 1967). Further, these interviews may have been conducted by a psychiatrist who had no contact with the family during the child's illness; it is possible that very different results may be obtained when parents and interviewer develop a relationship throughout the course of the child's illness. It is unfortunately true to say that the results generally reflect the interests of the investigators. As noted by Lavigne and Burns (1981):

> Studies that emphasize how frequently adjustment failures occur do not include measures that might tap the parent's optimal functioning. Likewise studies that conclude that the parents are functioning well often do not include standardized measures to estimate the presence of parental psychopathology other than anxiety. (p. 344)

These types of criticisms have led to a call for more detailed and systematic study of families throughout the period of the child's illness, from diagnosis through to disease-free remission or death (Nagler, 1978; Susman et al., 1980).

Kupst et al. (1982) studied 64 families from diagnosis for a 1-year period. The families were assessed using self-reports, ratings by physicians and nurses on family reactions and behavior in hospital, and ratings by psychosocial staff based on interviews. Parents also completed the California Psychological Inventory (Gough, 1964) and the Summed Coping Scale of this inventory. Both parents also completed the Current Adjustment Rating Scale (Berzins, Bednar, & Severy, 1975) at diagnosis, early outpatient treatment, later outpatient treatment, readmission (if applicable), after the death of the child (if applicable), and at the end of the study.

Medical staff rated the families on the Family Coping Scale (Hurwitz, Kaplan, & Kaiser, 1962). In addition, psychosocial staff rated families on the following antecedent variables: (1) previous course of the illness (few or none vs. complications), (2) medical status at 1 year (doing well vs. not doing well), (3) family intactness and quality of relationship, (4) adequacy of support system, (5) concurrent stresses, (6) sibling problems, and (7) financial problems. Psychosocial staff also noted the predominant coping behaviors of families at 1 year. These included information seeking, intrapsychic response (denial, anxiety, intellectualization), direct action (activity, humor, overprotectiveness, self-reliance), and inhibition of action (somatic complaints, use of drugs or alcohol, guilt, regressive behavior).

One of the most significant findings was that mothers reported themselves as coping better at 1-year postdiagnosis than on referral. There were no differences, however, between how physicians and psychosocial workers rated family coping on the two occasions. There was a high degree of correlation between how individual family members coped. Families of older children appeared to cope somewhat better than families of younger children.

Kupst et al. (1982) also attempted to identify those antecedent variables that might predict how well families coped. It was reported that the previous course of the illness was not related to coping, but family or marital problems were. Of the 15 families who were not coping well at 1 year, 60% had family problems, while only 24% of those who were coping well had family problems. At the same time families with additional high levels of stress (including financial problems or pregnancies) were coping poorly. For fathers, higher occupational status and good relationships with their wives were indicative of better coping. These data are interpreted as evidence that most families do cope reasonably well 1 year after diagnosis. The implication would be that despite the very aggressive nature of leukemia treatment and the constant uncertainty about the child's future, relatively normal lives can be led by families during periods of remission.

As Kupst et al. (1982) acknowledged, however, there are some problems in accepting these data. Some of the raw data were missing. Psychosocial staff planned to visit families in their homes at 1 year postdiagnosis, but in practice, "many families were involved in their own activities and tended to put off the home visits" (p. 171). If nurses and physicians did not feel able to rate coping behavior of families, they did not do so. This in itself may account for the apparent finding that fathers with higher economic status jobs were coping better than those in less prestigious employment. Finally, there is always the reservation that the instruments employed were not sensitive enough to pick up subtle effects of the disease.

Conclusions

Leukemia is such an obviously traumatic illness that there is a general recognition that many professionals—psychiatrists, psychologists, social workers, nursing and medical personnel—all have a key role to play to ensure the survival of the family. To date, there has been considerable work describing the adverse social effects on family life and adverse intellectual effects on the child. Considerably less attention has been paid to devising methods to alleviate family stress or reduce the impact of treatment on the child's mental development.

In the United States, special pediatric oncology nurses have been appointed at some major treatment centers (Greene, 1975); these nurses have been trained especially to deal with problems encountered by these families. Other researchers have reported on the potential usefulness of group sessions to enable parents to meet and share their concerns (Lansdown, 1980). For children, the most pressing practical need is to assist the return and integration into school (Greene, 1975; Katz, Kellerman, Rigler, Williams, & Siegel, 1977). One of the most debated questions is concerned with the extent to which the child should be informed about the disease and its treatment. The complexity of such a decision is sadly not reflected in any flurry of research interest. Few have directly approached the issue. Yet work by Slavin et al. (1982) suggests that early and honest communication about leukemia is a determinant of subsequent psychiatric and psychological adjustment. This study was, however, retrospective, and it would be useful to know a child's *immediate* reaction to this kind of news in addition to the long-term consequences. It is perhaps naive to assume that there is a single answer to the dilemma of what to tell the leukemic patient. Variations in personality of the patient and communicative style of the informant are likely to be critical also. Researchers have tended to avoid investigating problems of communication about cancer, precisely because it is a very difficult subject. Communication between parent and child can be difficult normally; studies such as those by Mulhern et al. (1981) highlight how such difficulties are compounded where the child has leukemia. Yet this research is very valuable, especially in highlighting how differently pediatrician, parent, and child view the situation. Mulhern et al. (1981) emphasize how the different parties weight information to arrive at their diverse estimates of the child's prognosis. The implications of this research are twofold: first, showing how misunderstandings between medical staff and the families can arise and second, pointing to those factors that families appear unable or unwilling to take into account. Physicians should probably realize that some parents will be reluctant to recognize many unsavory facts, however full the explanation that is given.

Unlike the situation with diabetes, there are no data on which any decisions could be taken about what to tell the child with leukemia. Account needs to be taken, however, of developmental changes in the child's understanding of illness generally and death and dying more specifically (Koocher, 1981). Unlike diabetes, leukemia does not involve the child in developing a repertoire of behaviors aimed at self-care. While there have been some attempts to describe the aspects of diabetes treatment that children of different ages are likely to understand (Johnson et al., 1982) there are no such similar guidelines for dealing with the leukemic child. Yet the very complexity involved suggests that such an approach may be called for. The child with leukemia must be subject to a great deal of investigation by medical personnel and be willing to swallow large quantities of medicine. Changes in the child's understanding of the role of medical personnel (Brewster, 1982) and reasons for medication (Bush, Iannotti, & Davidson, 1983) are therefore central. A child's resistance to medical procedures or medication needs to be handled within such a developmental context.

Appendix

Questionnaire Used by Levenson et al. (1983) to Compare Parents' and Children's Perceptions About Cancer

I. Responses to Tests and Treatments
   1. Are you afraid of the tests and treatments at this clinic?
      1. No, not at all afraid   2. A little afraid   3. Fairly afraid
      4. Very afraid
   2. How often do you understand why you are having these tests and treatments?
      1. Always   2. Usually   3. Rarely   4. Never
   3. How uncomfortable have these tests and treatments made you feel?
      1. Not uncomfortable at all   2. A little   3. Quite   4. Extremely
   4. How much choice have you had in the treatments you have received?
      1. Complete choice   2. Some choice   3. Very little choice
      4. No choice
   5. Do you feel that the amount of choice you have had has been
      1. Too much   2. Just right   3. Not enough

II. Need to Know Items (Responses ranged from 1—extremely important—to 4—unimportant)
   1. The effects of cancer and its treatment on my future appearance
   2. How I can help most with my treatment
   3. How my treatments help me
   4. What causes cancer
   5. What I can do to aid my future health
   6. How cancer will affect my career, social life, and marriage
   7. How my illness will affect other family members
   8. Ways I can talk to my friends and relatives about my illness
   9. The kinds of physical activities I can do
   10. What to expect if cancer spreads
   11. How my illness might affect my health later on
   12. The effects of alcohol, smoking or drugs on my illness
   13. How I can help pay medical bills
   14. What to do if I forget to take my medicine

*From "Disparities in disease-related perceptions of adolescent cancer patients and their parents" by P.M. Levenson, D.R. Copeland, J.R. Morrow, B. Pfefferbaum and Y. Silberberg, 1983, *Journal of Pediatric Psychology, 8*(1). Reprinted by permission of Plenum Press, 1983.

III. Responses Evoked by Information
  1. Does finding out more information about your illness usually make you want to
     1. Cooperate more with treatment plan
     2. Cooperate less with treatment plan
  2. How often do you ask someone directly about the things that are really bothering you?
     1. Always   2. Often   3. Rarely   4. Never
  3. When something unpleasant is going to happen to you do you like to know about it
     1. As soon as possible   2. Somewhat ahead of time
     3. Just before it happens   4. Not at all
  4. How often do you think about your illness?
     1. All of the time   2. Most of the time   3. Some of the time
     4. Very little   5. Never
IV. Additional Information
  1. Would it be helpful to you to have some more information about your illness now?
     1. Yes   2. No
  2. Would it be helpful if your family had more information about your illness?
     1. Yes   2. No
  3. Would it be helpful to you if your friend/teachers had more information about your illness?
     1. Yes   2. No

9

Toward a Synthesis

A Developmental Theory of Illness Behavior

In the introduction to this book, I reviewed previous theoretical approaches to understanding how chronic illness affects children and their families. Two major approaches were contrasted: the social psychological approach adopted by Wright (1960) and the more cognitive approach adopted by Lipowski (1970) and Mattson (1972). Subsequently, Pless and Pinkerton (1975) attempted to draw together the key components of both these models.

Attempts to test these models empirically have been incomplete. While they remain little more than a listing of the various factors that might be involved in an individual's response to any illness, some components of the models are likely to remain doggedly aloof from empirical investigation. In this context, variables such as the child's premorbid personality or family relationships prior to the illness are pertinent. Other variables may be somewhat easier to investigate. Lipowski (1970), for example, lists a number of disease-related variables that may influence response to illness. These include variables such as chronicity, severity, or how life-threatening or physically restricting the disease may be. While previous approaches of this kind have identified a large number of variables that may be relevant in predicting outcome, in many instances they have failed to specify the direction of any association between variable and outcome. For example, severity of disease has been identified as important; the initial assumption being that the more severe the disease, the poorer the likely outcome. Even within a single disease, however, there is rarely an agreed medical definition of what constitutes a "severe" form of the illness.

Asthma is perhaps the classic example. Age at onset, duration of treatment, number of attacks per year, or functional indices of airways obstructions have all been cited in definitions of severity (Williams & McNicol, 1975). Such empirical work as there is does not support the view that poorer psychological outcome is necessarily associated with more severe forms of an illness. Working with children with congenital heart defects, for example, both Garson et al. (1978) and Linde et al. (1966) suggest that milder forms of the disease are often associated with worse adjustment. Similarly, blind children have been reported to be better adjusted than those with partial visual impairments (Cowen et al., 1961), and deaf children have been reported to be better adjusted than those who are hard-of-hearing (Rodda, 1970; Sussman, 1966; Williams 1970). McFie and Robertson (1973) concluded that children more severely disabled as a result of the thalidomide drug were better adjusted than those with less serious disabilities. This all implies the possibility of a curvilinear relationship between severity of illness and adjustment, rather than a simple linear effect.

If it is difficult to quantify "severity" in relation to a single illness or disability, it is even more uncertain how one would attempt any comparison of different diseases in terms of severity. Since diseases vary along more than one dimension, empirical investigations are likely to be complicated. Nevertheless, research involving more than one disease is necessary to clarify how different characteristics of illnesses contribute to psychological reactions.

A Summary of the Cognitive Approach to Understanding Children's Concepts of Illness

The basic assumption behind this work is that children's ideas about health and illness develop in an ordered sequence, parallel to the acquisition of more physical concepts such as space or time. Thus, the stages described by Piaget (1970) as characterizing the child's thought in such physical concepts are also applicable to the understanding of bodily processes and causes and prevention of illness. Children's thought is thus believed to progress through the classic stages of prelogical, concrete-logical and formal-logical thought, with the main distinction between the three stages being the degree of differentiation made by the child between the self and others.

During the preoperational phase (2–7 years of age), Piaget believed that children were unable to reason beyond their immediate experiences. Children believed that things are as they seem, rather than as they must logically be. They are unable to take another person's viewpoint and are embedded in their own egocentric points of view. Thus, when faced with a three-dimensional visual display they assume that all perspectives will be identical with their own (Piaget & Inhelder, 1956). When asked to draw the inside of the body, the preoperational child has difficulty and tends to confuse internal and external parts. Beliefs about the inside of the body are limited by the child's assumption that the body contains only items that the child placed there. The preschooler typically draws items of food inside the body. Body parts drawn are limited to those such as bones that the child can feel or blood, which may be visible when the child cuts a finger. Beliefs about body functioning are also elementary. The child has no idea about how different parts are connected or about transformations occurring within the body. Thus, at this stage there is no conception of food being transformed into other substances and circulated round the body.

Concepts of illness are also naive. Early research concluded that young children perceived illness as a punishment (Langford, 1948), and even more recent work suggests that this belief is still common among some groups of children (Brewster, 1982). At this stage, children define illness in terms of its behavioral effects; "being ill" is equated with having to stay in bed. Conversely, "getting better" is synonomous with staying in bed and doing as the doctor says (Perrin & Gerrity, 1981). Children do not believe that anything can be done to prevent illness. Parallel with their belief that illness is a punishment, children also suspect that medical treatment is a form of punishment (Steward & Steward, 1981).

A major advance in cognitive development between 7 and 10 years of age enables the child to distinguish more clearly between what is internal and external in relation to the self. During this *concrete-operational* phase, children are able to use elementary logic, although thought is still limited by the child's own concrete experiences. In drawing their bodies, children do not confuse internal and external parts. However, the actual number of body parts known is still relatively small. Children are able to draw some major organs, such as the heart, brain, lungs and stomach, in approximately correct positions. They become aware of some of the transformations occurring within the body, for example, that food can be converted into blood, and circulated round the body. Simple explanations of the function of different organs occur. They know that the brain is needed for higher mental processes, but children at this stage are less sure about its role in more physical activities (Johnson & Wellman, 1982). Concepts of illness also become more differentiated. Children are aware that illness can be caused by germs (Bibace & Walsh, 1981), but they are confused about the precise mechanisms whereby illness is transferred across individuals. At around 9 years of age, children become aware that illness can be prevented.

At the most mature level of reasoning, Piaget (1930) describes a stage of *formal-operational* thought. Children are then capable of abstract thought and conceptualizing unseen objects and phenomena. They also understand physiological explanations of illness and can appreciate that immediate, unpleasant effects of treatment can be outweighed by long-term benefits. The child's knowledge of body anatomy and physiology is, in theory at least, complex and mature. Even among teenage groups, however, there is a suggestion that knowledge of reproductive organs and systems is poor (Gellert, 1962). The child well understands that substances can be transformed within the body and that illness can be caused by an interaction between enviromental substances and an individual vulnerability.

Criticisms of the Cognitive-Developmental Approach to Understanding Children's Beliefs About Illness

At a theoretical level, many criticisms and reservations can be made about work conducted so far. Although in his writings Piaget (1970) stressed that intelligence developed through the child's progressive adaptations to the environment, he did not investigate specifically the process of cognitive development as a function of environmental differences. More recent work has tended to stress far more the role of social interactions in influencing cognitive development (Light, 1983). While it has been recognized and demonstrated that social interactions can influence acquisition of purely cognitive concepts such as those involved in conservation tasks (Mugny, Perret-Clermont, & Doise, 1981; Perret-Clermont, 1980), there has been only speculation about the potentially greater role of social factors in influencing the child's development of health and illness concepts. Social and intrafamilial factors have been implicated by Mechanic (1964), Pratt (1973), and Neligan and Prudham (1974). It has also been hypothesized that the experience of illness itself will influence concepts of health and illness held by children. Predictions based on a purely cognitive theory of development would be that the experience of chronic illness would accelerate children's attainment of these concepts (Bibace & Walsh, 1981). Empirical work suggests that this is not the case (Caradang et al., 1979; Eiser, Patterson, & Tripp, 1984b; Simeonsson et al., 1979). This aspect of the work, too, has practical implications. Research so far does not indicate that there is any justification for assuming that a sick child will necessarily be at the same stage of understanding illness concepts as a healthy child of similar chronological age. However, almost without exception, research into the development of children's ideas about health and illness have been based on work with healthy children. In his criticisms of this work, Blos (1978) noted the irony of this situation, and stressed the need to investigate sick children's understanding of both health and illness concepts. Such criticisms can still be directed at the current research literature.

A third point to be made is that no research has been directed at the question of whether children's concepts of their bodies, health, and illness can be categorized in the same general stage of cognitive development. Thus, although it has been shown that the attainment of these concepts individually follow a Piagetian sequence, there are no data investigating the relationship between them. Thus, we do not know of the relationship between the development of the child's concepts of health, illness, and the body.

Bibace and Walsh (1981) consider briefly how the child's concepts of illness relate to development in more physical spheres. Some investigators have included measures of the child's concepts of physical phenomena in addition to those involving health and illness, (cf., Perrin & Gerrity, 1981).

The conclusions of these studies are that knowledge of health and illness lags behind that of physical phenomena. Crider (1981) tried to get round this difficulty by suggesting that the term "stage" should be dropped in favor of a term such as level of conceptualization. Koocher (1981) suggests that the only solution to the problem is to conduct longitudinal studies of the development of the child's thought. Scalogram analyses of the health concepts, comparable to those conducted with the child's concept of space for example, (Laurendeau & Pinard, 1970) would be a logical next step.

Implications for the Care of Sick Children

Notwithstanding these criticisms, it is apparent that there are many situations in pediatric medicine when interventions based on theoretical rather than intuitive grounds would be desirable. Not least it is apparent that such a schema can be used as a framework both to understand sick children's behavior and to address those specific aspects of the illness or its treatment that cause most concern.

The dilemma about what to tell the pediatric patient is of perhaps most obvious relevance. Whenever assessments of patients' knowledge about illness have been made, it has been demonstrated that both the quantity and quality of information has been poor. In the case of phenylketonuria, no systematic attempts to assess the child's understanding have been made. Assessments of parents have indicated that their own understanding is poor (Wood et al., 1967).

In diabetes, knowledge of both patients and parents has consistently been shown to be insufficient to enable everyday care to take place (cf., Johnson et al., 1982). Patients with asthma know little about their disease and do not understand how behaviors such as smoking can adversely affect their health (Martin et al., 1982). In leukemia, there is general recognition of the complexities involved in discussing the disease with a patient, yet there is little research effort directed at the question (Slavin et al., 1982). Parents of epileptic children are confused

about the implications of such a diagnosis for behavior and achievements (Ward & Bower, 1978) and such confusions color child-rearing
practices. In a study of parents of children with congenital heart disease,
Garson et al. (1978) concluded that only a small proportion had an
adequate understanding of the child's illness. Such widespread ignor-
ance cannot be totally attributable to a failure of medical personnel to
try to inform patients and their families, but suggests perhaps that the
kind of information given does not address itself to patients' own
informational needs. The following schema is a rough guide to
understanding developmental stages in the thoughts and behaviors of
the sick child.

It is acknowledged that children in the prelogical stage of thought
typically believe that illness is a punishment for misbehavior or perhaps
the result of magic. It would follow that the way to get better is to start
behaving. Chronically sick children in this age-range would therefore
be expected to be "good" patients and to conform with adult
instructions. For this group of children, accepting their illness is likely
to mean accepting their punishment or treatment. By the same token,
they are likely to make the inference that good health can be attained
just by doing as they are told and are not likely to feel that they have any
personal control over the outcome. We might also speculate about how
inferences of this kind might affect the child's general behavior.
Children are likely to expect that other punishments will be meeted out
for other misdemeanors, resulting in behavior that is unnaturally docile
and submissive.

Children in the concrete-logical stage of development understand
that illness is caused by infection from others. During this stage, too,
they begin to understand that illness can be prevented. While children
in the prelogical stage of thought believed that various body organs
functioned generally to keep them alive or well, children at the
concrete-logical stage of thought begin to differentiate organs and their
function. As a result of these changes in cognition, the understanding
and acceptance of personal illness of children in this stage is likely to be
qualitatively different from that of the preschooler. Children at this
stage overgeneralize about illness (Kister & Patterson, 1980), believing
that noncontagious illnesses are in fact infectious. This may lead to the
child avoiding others to prevent further illnesses being transmitted. The
chronically sick child of this age-group is thus very likely to become a
social isolate. The child's understanding of illness is also likely to be
colored by this belief and may lead to a greater questioning about the
value of other aspects of medical treatment.

At around 11 years of age, there supposedly emerges the beginning
of mature, adult reasoning. Children understand that illness can be
caused by different agents and that individuals can be differentially
vulnerable because of physiological or psychological factors. There is a
tendency to assume that once this stage has been reached, acceptance of

the disease and adherence to treatment should follow. In fact, the evidence that there is suggests that it is during adolescence that real rebellion to treatment and medical personnel is most likely. Perhaps we should not be surprised at this. An adult understanding of illness involves recognizing the arbitrary nature of becoming ill. Having just mastered the concept of illness prevention, the child is immediately faced with the fact that personal illness is often caused for no good reason, and no personal action could have prevented it. The implications are that the child needs to work through these inconsistencies. It is only at this stage that individual differences in variables such as locus of control are likely to have any implication for illness behavior. In understanding that there is a personal element in combating disease, variables such as locus of control may become relevant in determining adolescent behavior.

In summary, a developmental approach to chronic illness needs to allow for the fact that the child's beliefs about why the illness occurred, what needs to be done to prevent a reoccurrence, and how it is to be cured differ markedly from the adult view. This needs to be taken account of at both a practical and theoretical level. At a practical level, the work has some implications for dealing with sick children. The question is especially important for children in the so-called prelogical stage of thought.

It should be remembered that some 50% of under 7-year-olds will be admitted to hospital (Davie et al., 1972) and that children between 7 months and 4 years of age are apparently highly vulnerable in this situation (Rachman & Phillips, 1975). There is consequently a real need to develop adequate guidelines for communicating with sick children and understanding their behavior. Bibace and Walsh (1981) do make some suggestions as to the kind of information about hospitalization that would be suitable for this age-group. Explanations, they suggest, should be very practical in nature, focusing on descriptions of medical equipment or differences between nursing staff in terms of their uniform. Both Johnson et al. (1982) and Harkavy et al. (1983) propose that explanations of diabetes should be limited to information about the child's diet, rather than including details about insulin or urine tests. The restricted cognitive level of this age-group means that information must be very simple and concrete.

It is apparent that children between the ages of 7 and 11 years are cognitively able to understand a much wider range of issues than children less than 7 years. Children's understanding is nevertheless enhanced where explanations draw on their own experiences. Several researchers have advocated the potential use of metaphors in explaining illness to the child. Whitt, Dykstra, and Taylor (1979) give several examples. Epilepsy, for example, might be explained by likening the brain to a telephone that sends messages to all parts of the body. The brain can call up a finger to move, a foot to kick, a mouth to talk, and so on. Seizures can be likened to a telephone getting a wrong number. Just like a telephone, after the wrong number the phone number works fine again and the brain, too, can send messages to the body just as needed.

Other metaphors that might be used to explain nephrotic syndrome, cancer, or hydrocephalus are also given by Whitt et al. (1979). Nephrotic syndrome, for example, and diabetes can be explained in terms of failure on the part of the body to equate energy input with actual requirements. Medical treatment therefore involves additional calls at the "garage for refueling." Cancer is explained by likening the body to a large city. In a city, it can be explained, there are many people all with different but vital jobs to do. In the same way the body is composed of many different cells, each with their own vital function. Cancer is then the result of some of the cells adopting an "outlaw" role and attacking the legitimate cells. Treatment may then be presented as a means of supplementing the body's own police force and exterminating the outlaws. Beales et al. (1983) speculate that an adequate explanation of arthritis for the 7- to 11-year-old child might involve likening blood vessels to pipelines and nerves to electric wiring. Further explanations might involve suggesting that the body's defending army has been incompetent at identifying the enemy and has turned on itself instead.

During the stage of formal-operational thought, there is a belief that children's essentially physiological understanding of illness means that they can understand medical explanations of illness and accept the short-term discomfort of treatment in the knowledge that long-term relief will occur.

Schemata such as these have definite intuitive appeal. Yet supporting evidence is scarce, and it would be premature to assume that problems in communicating with sick children were negligible. It is not clear that adults, let alone adolescents, understand physiological explanations of illness (Ley, 1982). At the same time, it is not clear that children in the concrete-logical stage of thought do find it easier to understand explanations of illness in terms of nonmedical analogies rather than medical terms. Whitt et al. (1979) warn that care needs to be taken in this respect. Certainly some investigation of how children understand such analogies and the inferences they draw for other aspects of illness and treatment is essential. A too literal interpretation of some analogies may be potentially more damaging than no explanation at all.

Implications for Dealing With the Parents of Sick Children

I have discussed at length the repercussions of chronic illness on the child's intellectual, social, and personality development. I have also attempted to describe the implications of this work for understanding the behavior of sick children. Equally, it is important to realize that this research has implications for helping parents care for their sick children. Child rearing raises many problems under normal circumstances, but everyday dilemmas can assume greater significance when the child suffers from a chronic illness. Eating, for example, can be a source of conflict in any family. Where diet is implicated in the treatment of the disease, as in PKU or diabetes, for example, it is probable that greater conflict still will arise. Temper tantrums are an integral part of the behavior of most toddlers, and many parents are unsure of how to cope with tantrums even when their child is healthy. Ward and Bower (1978) have shown that some parents are afraid that temper tantrums may precipitate epileptic seizures. It would not be surprising if parents of diabetic children similarly feared that tantrums might lead to hypoglycemia attacks, in that parents generally are told to expect obstreperous behavior prior to such attacks. In either case, parents are likely to adopt very lenient approaches to child rearing. Markova, Stirling-Phillips, and Forbes (1984) have pointed out that parents of hemophiliac boys are anxious that the child may cut himself with sharp tools and bleed. They therefore tend to limit opportunity to play with knives and scissors. As a consequence, the boys are less experienced and more careless in their use of tools than healthy age-matched peers. These are all practical difficulties that parents do need advice on. In terms of managing their child, this sort of information is much more important than more theoretical ideas about the cause of illness and rationale for treatment.

It is less clear how far it is desirable to alert parents to the potentially adverse effects of chronic illness documented in the literature. On the whole, it does not seem justifiable to alert all parents of sick children that such difficulties might be encountered. Ward and Bower (1978) report that even for parents of children with epilepsy and normal intelligence, there is considerable anxiety that the child might be retarded. Parents look for signs to indicate that some mental deterioration is developing. Any warning to parents of children with other illnesses that some compromise in mental development is possible is likely to result in similar anxiety. In that research has failed to identify those children who are most likely to suffer intellectual or social consequences of a disease, there seems little reason to alert *all* parents to such a possibility. Not all children react to illness in this way, and researchers have hardly begun to determine the characteristics of those who are most vulnerable.

Perhaps, though, the information should be of use in educational settings. Teachers are far from confident in dealing with sick children (Fitzherbert, 1982). They often know very little about the complaint and are worried about what to do if the child becomes ill in school. Bradbury and Smith (1983) for example reported that only 24% of 97 teachers of diabetic pupils had an adequate understanding of diabetes.

Isolated reports of attempts to improve communication with hospital and school have all apparently met with success (Farquhar & Campbell, 1980; Katz et al., 1977). An integral part of teacher training schemes should ideally include some directives for dealing with sick children. At the very least, misinformed stereotypes about the behavior of the chronically sick need to be dispelled (Weinberg & Santana, 1978).

Summary

There has been a great deal of work attempting to describe the social effects of chronic childhood illness on the child and family. Much of this rests on the assumption that illness must adversely affect the development of the child and interactions within the family. With regard to the development of the child, there is evidence that some compromise in intellectual, personal, and social development takes place. With regard to the family, there is evidence of increased marital stress and divorce and greater psychological conflict over child care. It would not be accurate to suggest that all work in this tradition was equally pessimistic about the prognosis for child and family, but it certainly is representative of a large proportion of the work. It has been observed by previous writers (Pless & Pinkerton, 1975) that the work in this area lacks cohesion or direction, and this has been attributed to a lack of a theoretical framework around which research can be oriented. While earlier theories (Lipowski, 1970; Wright, 1960) have been commendable in the degree to which they have tabulated variables that might influence attitudes to illness, they have been less successful in relating these together. Any attempts that have been made tend to be ad hoc. Thus it is all very well to expect that age of diagnosis is an important variable, but it is more difficult to predict *how* age affects the child. Certainly there is no simple linear relationship.

A quite distinct body of work has developed concerned with describing how the child's knowledge of illness and illness related concepts (causes, prevention, treatment) change during childhood. This work was reviewed in Chapter 2. Although it has been made clear that this area of research needs a great deal of clarification, it is sufficiently established to be used as an adjunct to previous work on the development of chronically sick children.

The conclusions of this research are that the meaning of illness changes during childhood and cannot be understood purely in terms of arbitrary definitions extrapolated from adult views. Rather, the implications are that variations in psychological outcome are dependent on children's cognitive construction of the reasons for their illness and on their concomitant expectations for the future.

References

Aaron, N. S. (1967). Some personality differences between asthmatic, allergic and normal children. *Journal of Clinical Psychology, 23*, 336–340.

Aaronson, D. (1972). Asthma: General concepts. In R. Patterson (Ed.), *Allergic disease: Diagnosis and management* (pp. 197–239). Philadelphia: Lippincott.

Abramson, H. A. (1954). Evaluation of maternal rejection theory in allergy. *Annals of Allergy, 12*, 129–140.

Abroms, K. I., & Kodera, T. L. (1979). Acceptance hierarchy of handicaps: Validation of Kirk's statement, "Special education often begins where medicine stops." *Journal of Learning Disabilities, 12*, 15–20.

Ack, M., Miller, I., & Weil, W. B., Jr. (1961). Intelligence of children with diabetes mellitus. *Pediatrics, 28*, 764–770.

Acosta, P. B., Fiedler, J. L., & Koch, R. (1968). Mothers' dietary management of PKU children. *Journal of the American Dietetic Association, 53*, 460–464.

Agle, D. P. (1964). Psychiatric studies of patients with hemophilia and related states. *Archives of Internal Medicine, 144*, 76–82.

Ahlfield, J. E., Soler, N. G., & Marcus, S. D. (1983). Adolescent diabetes mellitus: Parent/child perspectives of the effect of the disease on family and social interactions. *Diabetes Care, 6*(4), 393–398.

Alcock, T. (1960). Some personality characteristics of asthmatic children. *Journal of Medical Psychology, 33*, 133–141.

Allan, J. L., Townley, R. R. W., & Phelan, R. D. (1974). Family response to cystic fibrosis. *Australian Paediatric Journal, 10*, 136–146.

Allen, D. W., & Cole, P. (1972). Viruses and human cancer. *New England Journal of Medicine, 286*, 70–82.

Allen, J. C. (1978). The effects of cancer on the nervous system. *Journal of Pediatrics, 93*, 903–909.

Allen, R. J., & Gibson, R. M. (1961). Phenylketonuria with normal intelligence. *American Journal of Diseases of Children, 102*, 115–122.

Alogna, M. (1980). Perception of severity of disease and health locus of control in compliant and non-compliant diabetic patients. *Diabetes   Care, 3,* 533–534.

Anderson, H. R., Bailey, P. A., Cooper, J. S., Palmer, J. S., & West, S. (1983). Morbidity and school absence caused by asthma and wheezing illness. *Archives of Disease in Childhood, 58,* 777–784.

Apley, J., Barbour, R. F., & Westmacott, I. (1967). Impact of congenital heart disease on the family: Preliminary report. *British Medical Journal, 10,* 103–105.

Appelboom-Fondu, J., Verstraeten, F., & Van Loo-Reynaers, J. (1977). Comparative study of psychological aspects between diabetic and hemophilic children. In Z. Laron (Ed.), *Pediatric adolescent endocrinology: Vol. 3. Psychological aspects of balance of diabetes in juveniles.* Basel: Karger.

Auer, E. T., Senturia, A. G., & Shopper, M. (1971). Congenital heart disease and childhood adjustment. *International Journal of Psychiatry in Medicine, 2,* 23–30.

Azarnoff, P., & Woody, P. (1981). Preparation of children for hospitalization in acute care hospitals in the United States. *Pediatrics, 68*(3), 361–368.

Bacon, C. L. (1956). The role of aggression in the asthmatic attack. *Psychoanalytic Quarterly, 25,* 309–323.

Bagley, C. (1971). *The social psychology of the child with epilepsy.* Coral Gables, FL: University of Miami Press.

Baker, L., Minuchin, S., Milman, L., Leibman, R., & Todd, T. (1975). Psychosomatic aspects of juvenile diabetes mellitus. A progress report. In Z. Laron (Ed.), *Modern problems in pediatrics. Vol. 12. Diabetes in juveniles: Medical and rehabilitation aspects.* New York: Karger.

Baker, L., Rosman, B. L., Sargent, J., & Noguerira, J. (1982). *Family factors predict glycosylated hemoglobin in juvenile diabetes: A prospective study.* Paper presented at the meeting of the American Diabetes Association, San Francisco, CA.

Bandura, A., & Walters, R. (1963). *Social learning and personality development.* New York: Holt, Rinehart.

Barker, R. G., Wright, B., & Myerson, L. (1953) *Adjustment to physical handicap and illness: A survey of the social psychology of physique and disability.* New York: Social Science Research Council.

Barr, L. W., & Logan, G. B. (1964). Prognosis of children having asthma. *Pediatrics, 34,* 856–860.

Barsch, R. H. (1968). *The parent of the handicapped child.* Springfield, IL: C. C. Thomas.

Bastiaans, J., & Groen, J. (1955). Psychogenesis and psychotherapy of bronchial asthma. In D. O'Neill (Ed.), *Modern trends in psychosomatic medicine,* (pp. 242–268). London: Butterworth and Co.

Baumeister, A. A. (1967). The effects of dietary control on intelligence in phenylketonuria. *American Journal of Mental Deficiency, 71,* 840–847.

Beales, J. G., Holt, P. J. L., Keen, J. H., & Mellor, V. P. (1983). Children with juvenile chronic arthritis: Their beliefs about their illness and therapy. *Annals of the Rheumatic Diseases, 42,* 481–486.

Becker, R. D. (1972). Therapeutic approaches to psychopathological reactions to hospitalization. *International Journal of Child Psychotherapy, 1,* 65–97.

Beckwith, C., Cohen, S. E., Kopp, C. B., Parmelee, A. H., & Marcy, T. G. (1976).

Caregiver–infant interaction and early cognitive development in preterm infants. *Child Development, 47,* 579–587.

Beckwith, L., & Cohen, S. E. (1978). Preterm birth: Hazardous obstetrical and postnatal events as related to caregiver–infant behavior. *Infant Behavior and development, 1,* 1–14.

Beisser, A. R. (1979). Denial and affirmation in illness and health. *American Journal of Psychiatry, 136,* 1026–1030.

Bentovim, A. (1968). Controlled observations of phenylketonuric children on and during withdrawal from low phenylalanine diet. *Archives of Disease in Childhood, 43,* 745–746.

Bergmann, T., & Freud, A. (1965). *Children in the hospital.* New York: International Press.

Berman, P. W., Graham, F. K., Eichman, P. L., & Waisman, H. A. (1961). Psychologic and neurologic status of diet-treated phenylketonuric children and their siblings. *Pediatrics, 28,* 924–934.

Berman, P. W., Waisman, H. A., & Graham, F. K. (1966). Intelligence in phenylketonuric children—A developmental study. *Child Development, 37,* 731–747.

Berry, H. K., O'Grady, D. J., Perlmutter, M. K., & Bofinger, M. K. (1979). Intellectual development and academic achievement of children treated early for phenlketonuria. *Developmental Medicine and Child Neurology, 21,* 311–320.

Berzins, J. I., Bednar, R. L., & Severy, L. J. (1975). The problem of intersource consensus in measuring therapeutic outcomes: New data and multivariate perspectives. *Journal of Abnormal Psychology, 84,* 10–19.

Beverley, B. (1936). The effect of illness upon emotional development. *Journal of Pediatrics, 8* (May), 533–543.

Bialer, I. (1961). Conceptualization of success and failure in mentally retarded and normal children. *Journal of Personality, 29,* 303–320.

Bibace, R., & Walsh, M. E. (1980). Development of children's concepts of illness. *Pediatrics, 66,* 913–917.

Bibace, R., & Walsh, M. E. (1981). Children's conceptions of illness. In R. Bibace & M. E. Walsh (Eds.), *New Directions for Child Development* (pp. 31–48). (Vol. 14). San Francisco: Jossey-Bass.

Bickel, H. (1980). Phenylketonuria: Past, present, and future. F. P. Hudson Memorial Lecture, Leeds, 1979. *Journal of Inherited Metabolic Disease, 3*(4), 123–132.

Bickel, H., Gerrard, J., & Hickmans, E. M. (1954). The influence of phenylalanine intake on the chemistry and behaviour of a phenylketonuric child. *Acta Paediatrica Scandinavica 43,* 64–77.

Bidder, R. T., Crowe, E. A., & Gray, O. P. (1974). Mothers' attitudes to preterm infants. *Archives of Disease in Childhood, 49,* 766–770.

Binger, C. M. (1973). Childhood leukemia—Emotional impact on siblings. In E. J. Anthony & C. Koupernick (Eds.), *The child in his family: Vol. 2. The impact of disease and death* (pp. 195–210). New York: Wiley.

Binger, C. M., Ablin, A. R., Feuerstein, R. C., Kushner, J. H., Zoger, S., & Mikkelson, C. (1969). Childhood leukemia: Emotional impact on patient and family. *New England Journal of Medicine, 280,* 414–418.

Blair, H. (1977). Natural history of childhood asthma: Twenty year follow-up. *Archives of Disease in Childhood, 52,* 613–619.

Blinder, B. J. (1972). Sibling death in childhood. *Child Psychiatry and Human Development, 2,* 169–175.

Blos, P. (1978). Children think about illness: Their conceptual beliefs. In E. Gellert (Ed.), *Psychosocial aspects of pediatric care* (pp. 1–17). New York: Grune & Stratton.

Blum, L. H. (1977). Health information via mass media: Study of the individual's concepts of the body and its parts. *Psychological Reports, 40,* 991–999.

Boyce, W. T., Jensen, E. W., Cassel, J. C., Collier, A. M., Smith, A. H., & Ramey, C. T. (1977). Influence of life events and family routines on childhood respiratory tract illness. *Pediatrics, 60*(4),1 609–615.

Boyle, C. M. (1970). Differences between doctors' and patients' interpretations of some common medical terms. *British Medical Journal, 2,* 286–289.

Boyle, I. R., di Sant'Agnese, P., Sack, S., Millican, F., & Kukzycki, L. L. (1976). Emotional adjustment of adolescents and young adults with cystic fibrosis. *Journal of Pediatrics, 88,* 318–326.

Bowlby, J. (1952). *Maternal care and mental health* (2nd ed.). Geneva, Switzerland: World Health Organisation Monograph, No. 2.

Bozeman, M. F., Orbach, C. E., & Sutherland, A. M. (1955). The adaptation of mothers to the threatened loss of their child through leukemia. *Cancer, 8,* 1–33.

Bradbury, A. J., & Smith, C. S. (1983). An assessment of the diabetic knowledge of school teachers. *Archives of Disease in Childhood, 58,* 692–696.

Brain, D. J., & Maclay, I. (1968). Controlled study of mothers and children in hospital. *British Medical Journal* [Clinical Research Ed.] *1,* 278–280.

Brazelton, T. B., Holder, R., & Talbot, B. (1953). Emotional aspects of rheumatic fever in children. *Journal of Pediatrics, 63,* 339–358.

Brewster, A. B. (1982). Chronically ill hospitalized children's concepts of their illness. *Pediatrics, 69,* 355–362.

Brieland, D. (1967). A follow-up study of orthopedically handicapped high school graduates. *Exceptional Children, 33,* 555.

Brodie, B. (1974). Views of healthy children toward illness. *American Journal of Public Health, 64,* 1156–1159.

Bronheim, S. P. (1978). Pulmonary disorders: Asthma and cystic fibrosis. In P. R. Magreb (Ed.), *Psychological management of pediatric problems: Vol. 1. Early life conditions and chronic diseases* (pp. 309–321). Baltimore: University Park Press.

Brown, G. D., & Thompson, W. H. (1940). The diabetic child: An analytic study of his development. *American Journal of Diseases of Children, 59,* 238–254.

Brown, J. V., & Bakeman, R. (1979). Relationships of human mothers with their infants during the first year of life. In R. W. Bell & W. P. Smotherman (Eds.), *Maternal influences and early behavior.* Holliswood, NY: Spectrum.

Bruch, H. (1948). Physiologic and psychologic interrelationships in diabetes in children. *Psychosomatic Medicine, 11,* 200–210.

Bruhn, J. G. (1977). Self-concept and the control of diabetes. *American Family Physician, 15,* 93–97.

Bruhn, J. G., Hampton, J. W., & Chandler, B. C. (1971). Clinical marginality and psychological adjustment in hemophilia. *Journal of Psychosomatic Research,* *15*, 207–213.

Brunner, R. L., Jordan, M. K., & Berry, H. K. (1983). Early-treated phenyl-ketonuria: Neuropsychologic consequences. *Journal of Pediatrics, 102,* 831–835.

Buist, N. R., Lis, E. W., Tuerck, J. M., & Murphy, W. H. (1979). Maternal phenylketonuria. *Lancet, 2,* 589.

Burstein, S., & Meichenbaum, D. (1979). The work of worrying in children undergoing surgery. *Journal of Abnormal Child Psychology, 7,* 121–132.

Burton, L. (1975). *The family life of sick children.* London: Routledge and Kegan Paul.

Bush, P. J., Iannotti, R. J., & Davidson, F. R. (1983). *A children's health behavior model and expectations to take medicine.* Unpublished manuscript, Georgetown University School of Medicine, Washington, D.C.

Butler, N. (1980). Child health and education in the seventies: Some results on the 5-year follow-up of the 1970 British Birth Cohort. *Health Visitor, 35,* 81–82.

Byler, R., & Lewis, G. (1969). *Teach us what we want to know.* New York: Mental Health Materials Center.

Cabalska, B., Duczynska, N., Borzymowska, J., Zorska, K., Koślacz-Folga, A., & Bozkowa, K. (1977). Termination of dietary treatment in PKU. *European Journal of Pediatrics, 126,* 253–262.

Cain, A. C., Fast, I., & Erikson, M. E. (1964). Children's disturbed reactions to death of sibling. *American Journal of Orthopsychiatry, 34,* 741–752.

Calnan, M., & Peckham, C. S. (1977). Incidence of insulin-dependent diabetes in the first sixteen years of life. *Lancet, 1,* 589–590.

Campbell, J. D. (1975). Illness is a point of view: The development of children's concepts of illness. *Child Development, 46,* 92–100.

Caplan, G. (1961). *Prevention of mental disorders in children.* New York: Basic Books.

Caradang, M. L. A., Folkins, C. H., Hines, P. A., & Steward, M. S. (1979). The role of cognitive level and sibling illness in children's conceptualization of illness. *American Journal of Orthopsychiatry, 49,* 474–481.

Cassell, S., & Paul, M. (1967). The role of puppet therapy on the emotional responses of children hospitalized for cardiac catheterization. *Pediatrics, 71,* 233–239.

Cayler, G. C., Lynn, D. B., & Stein, E. M. (1973). Effect of cardiac "nondisease" on intellectual and perceptual motor development. *British Heart Journal, 35,* 543–547.

Centrewall, W. R., & Centrewall, C. (1961). Metabolic errors and mental retardation. *Clinical Medicine (Winnetka), 8,* 2109–2116.

Cernek, D., Hafner, G., Kos, S., & Cenlec, P. (1977). Comparative study of social and psychological analyses in asthmatic, rheumatic and diabetic children. *Allergie und Immunology, 23,* 214–220.

Chang, P. N., & Fisch, R. O. (1976). Observation of behavioral and personality characteristics to their dietary duration: Early treatment and normal intelligence. *Psychological Reports, 39,* 835–841.

Chessells, J. (1981). Acute leukaemia in childhood: Present problems and future prospects. In D. Hull (Ed.), *Recent advances in paediatrics* (pp. 157–178). Edinburgh & London: Churchill-Livingstone.

Chodoff, P., Friedman, S. B., & Hamburg, D. A. (1964). Stress, defenses and coping behavior: Observation in parents of children with malignant disease. *American Journal of Psychiatry, 120,* 743–749.

Clare, A. W., & Cairns, V. E. (1978). Design, development and use of a standardised interview to assess social maladjustment and dysfunction in community studies. *Psychological Medicine, 8,* 589–604.

Cobb, B. (1956). Psychological impact of long illness and death of a child on the family circle. *Journal of Pediatrics, 49,* 746–751.

Coddington, R. D. (1972). The significance of life events as etiologic factors in the diseases of children. *Journal of Psychosomatic Research, 16,* 7–18.

Cohen, S. I. (1971). Psychological factors in asthma: A review of their aetiolocial and therapeutic significance. *Postgraduate Medical Journal, 47,* 533–540.

Collier, B. N., & Etzwiler, D. D. (1971). Comparative study of diabetes knowledge among juvenile diabetics and their parents. *Diabetes, 20,* 51–57.

Collins, J. L. (1969). *Communication between deaf children of pre-school age and their mothers.* Unpublished doctoral dissertation, University of Pittsburgh.

Comaroff, J., & Maguire, P. (1981). Ambiguity and the search for meaning: Childhood leukaemia in the modern clinical context. *Social Science and Medicine, Part B, Medical Anthropology (Oxford). 15,* 115–123.

Conners, C. K. (1969). A teacher rating scale for use in drug studies with children. *American Journal of Child Psychiatry, 126,* 884–888.

Cook, S. D. (1975). *The development of causal thinking with regard to physical illness among French children.* Unpublished manuscript, University of Kansas, Lawrence, KS.

Coolidge, J. C. (1956). Asthma in mother and child as a special type of intercommunication. *American Journal of Orthopsychiatry, 26,* 165–178.

Cowen, E. L., Underberg, R. P., Verillo, R. T., & Benham, F. G. (1961). *Adjustment to visual disability in adolescence.* New York: American Foundation for the Blind.

Craig, O. (1982). *Childhood diabetes: The facts.* Oxford: Oxford University Press.

Crain, A. R., Sussman, M. B., & Weil, W. B. Jnr. (1966). Effects of a diabetic child on marital integration and related measures of family functioning. *Journal of Health and Human Behavior, 7,* 122–127.

Crider, C. (1981). Children's conceptions of the body interior. In R. Bibace & M. Walsh (Eds.), *New directions for child development: No. 14. Children's conceptions of health, illness and bodily functions* (pp. 49–66). San Francisco: Jossey Bass.

Cutter, F. (1955). *Maternal behavioir and childhood allergy.* Washington, D.C.: Catholic University of American Press.

Davie, R., Butler, N., & Goldstein, H. (1972) *From birth to seven.* London: Longmans.

Davis, D. M., Shipp, J. C., & Pattishall, E. G. (1965). Attitudes of diabetic boys and girls toward diabetes. *Diabetes, 14,* 106–109.

Davis, F. (1963). *Passage through crisis: Polio victims and their families.* Indianapolis, Ind.: Bobbs-Merrill.

Dekker, B., Barendregt, J., & de Vries, K. (1961). Allergy and neurosis in asthma. *Journal of Psychosomatic Research, 5*, 83–89.

Delbridge, L. (1975). Educational and psychological factors in the management of diabetes in childhood. *Medical Journal of Australia, 2*, 737–739.

Department of Health and Social Security, Office of Population and Census, Surveys, Welsh Office; Hospital In-Patient Enquiry (1979), Series MB4, No. 12, 1982.

Dikmen, S., Mathews, C. G., & Harley, J. P. (1975). The effect of early vs. late onset of major motor epilepsy upon cognitive intellectual performance. *Epilepsia, 16*, 73–81.

Dimock, H. G. (1960). *The child in hospital: A study of his emotional and social well-being.* Philadelphia: Davis.

Divitto, B., & Goldberg, S. (1979). The effects of newborn medical status on early parent–infant interaction. In T. Field, A. Sostek, S. Goldberg, H. H. Schuman (Eds.), *Infants born at risk* (pp. 311–331). New York: Spectrum.

Dobbing, J. (1968). Vulnerable periods in the developing brain. In A. N. Davidson & J. Dobbing (Eds.), *Applied neurochemistry* (pp. 287–316). Oxford: Blackwell.

Dobbing, J. (1974). The later development of the brain and its vulnerability. In J. A. Davis & J. Dobbing (Eds.), *Scientific foundations of paediatrics* (pp. 565–576). London: Heinemann Medical.

Dobson, J. C., Williamson, M. C., Azen, C., & Koch, R. (1977). Intellectual assessment of 111 4-year-old children with phenylketonuria. *Pediatrics, 60*, 822–827.

Donker, D. M., Reits, D., Storm, A., Van Leeuwen, L., Van Sprang, F. T., & Wadman, S. K. (1978). Computer analysis of the EEG as an aid in terminating diet therapy in PKU. *Revue d Electroencephalographie et de neurophysiologie Clinique (Paris), 8*, 55–60.

Douglas, J. (1975). Early hospital admissions and later disturbances of behaviour and learning. *Developmental Medicine and Child Neurology, 17*, 456–480.

Douglas, J. W. B., & Blomfield, J. M. (1958). *Children under five.* London, Allen & Unwin.

Downing, R. W., Moed, G., & Wright, B. (1961). Studies of disability: A technique for psychological measurement or effects. *Child Development, 32*, 561–575.

Dubo, S. (1950). Psychiatric study of children with pulmonary tuberculosis. *American Journal of Orthopsychiatry, 20* (July), 520–528.

Dubo, S., McLean, J. A., Ching, A. Y. T., Wright, H. L., Kauffman, P. E., & Sheldon, J. M. (1961). A study of relationships between family situation, bronchial asthma and personal adjustment in children. *Journal of Pediatrics, 59*, 402–414.

Dunbar, F. (1954). *Emotions and bodily changes.* New York: Columbia University Press.

Eggland, E. T. (1973). Locus of control and children with cerebral palsy. *Nursing Research, 22*, 329–333.

Ehrlich, R. M. (1974). Diabetes mellitus in childhood. In H. W. Bain (Ed.),

Pediatric clinics of North America: Vol. 21. Symposium on chronic disease in children (pp. 871–884). Philadelphia: W. B. Saunders.

Eiser, C. (1978). Intellectual abilities among survivors of childhood leukaemia as a function of CNS irradiation. *Archives of Disease in Childhood, 53*, 391–395.

Eiser, C. (1980a). The effects of chronic illness on intellectual development: A comparison of normal children with those treated for childhood leukaemia and solid tumours. *Archives of Disease in Childhood, 55*, 766–770.

Eiser, C. (1980b). How leukaemia affects a child's schooling. *British Journal of Social and Clinical Psychology, 19*, 365–368.

Eiser, C. (1981). Psychological sequelae of brain tumours in childhood: A retrospective study. *British Journal of Clinical Psychology, 20*, 35–38.

Eiser, C., & Lansdown, R. (1977). A retrospective study of intellectual development in children treated for acute lymphoblastic leukaemia. *Archives of Disease in Childhood, 52*, 525–529.

Eiser, C., & Patterson, D. (1983). "Slugs and snails and puppy-dog tails": Children's ideas about the insides of their bodies. *Child: Care, Health and Development, 9*, 233–240.

Eiser, C., Patterson, D., & Town, R. (in press). Knowledge of diabetes and implications for self-care. *Diabetic Medicine*.

Eiser, C., Patterson, D., & Eiser, J. R. (1983). Children's knowledge of health and illness: Implications for health education. *Child: Care, Health and Development, 9*, 285–292.

Eiser, C., Patterson, D., & Town, R. (1984). *Knowledge of diabetes and implications for self-care*. Manuscript submitted for publication.

Eiser, C., Patterson, D., & Tripp, J. H. (1984a). Diabetes and developing knowledge of the body. *Archives of Disease in Childhood, 59*, 167–169.

Eiser, C., Patterson, D., & Tripp, J. H. (1984b). Illness experience and children's conceptualisation of health and illness. *Child: Care, Health and Development, 10*, 157–162.

Eissler, R. S., Kris, M., & Solnitt, A. J. (1977). *Physical illness and handicap in childhood*. New Haven, CT: Yale University Press.

Elliot, C., Murray, D., & Pearson, L. (1978). *British ability scales*. Windsor, U.K.: NFER Publishing.

Ellis, E. F. (1975). Allergic disorders. In V. Vaughn, & R. J. McKay. (Eds.), *Nelson textbook of pediatrics* (pp. 492–521). Philadelphia: W. B. Saunders.

Epstein, L., Coburn, C., Becker, D., Drash, A., & Siminiero, L. (1980). Measurement and modification of the accuracy of determinations of urine glucose concentration. *Diabetes Care, 3*, 535–536.

Epstein, R. (1963, September). *Need for approval and the conditioning of verbal hostility in asthmatic children*. Paper presented at the meeting of the American Psychological Association, Philadelphia.

Erickson, E. H. (1940). Studies in the interpretation of play. 1. Clinical observations of play disruption in young children. *Genetic Psychology Monographs, 22*, 557–671.

Etzwiler, D. D. (1962). What the juvenile diabetic knows about his disease. *Pediatrics, 29*, 135–141.

Etzwiler, D., & Sines, L. (1962). Juvenile diabetes and its management: Family, social and academic implications. *Journal of the American Medical Association, 181*, 304–308.

Fallstrom, K. (1974). On the personality structure in diabetic school children. *Acta Paediatrica Scandinavica, 251* (Suppl.) 5–71.

Farber, B. (1959). Effects of a severely mentally retarded child on family integration. *Monographs of the Society for Research in Child Development, 24*(2, Serial No. 71).

Farber, B. (1960). Family organization and crisis: Maintenance of integration in families with a severely mentally retarded child. *Monographs of the Society for Research in Child Development, 25*(2, Serial No. 75).

Farquhar, J. W., & Campbell, M. L. (1980). Care of the diabetic child in the community. *British Medical Journal, 281*, 1534–1537.

Ferguson, B. F. (1979). Preparing young children for hospitalization: A comparison of two methods. *Pediatrics, 65*, 656–664.

Ferreira, A. J., & Winter, W. D. (1968). Information exchange and silence in normal and abnormal families. *Family Process, 5*, 60–75.

Field, T. M. (1977). Effects of early separation, interactive deficits, and experimental manipulations on mother–infant interaction. *Child Development, 48*, 763–771.

Fine, R. (1963). The personality of the asthmatic child. In H. I. Schneer (Ed.), *The asthmatic child: Psychosomatic approach to problems and treatment* (pp. 45–78). New York: Hoeber.

Fisch, R. O., Conley, J. A., Eysenbach, S., & Chang, P. (1977). Contact with phenylketonurics and their familes beyond pediatric age: Conclusions from a survey and conference. *Mental Retardation, 15*, 10–12.

Fischer, A. E., & Dolger, H. (1946). Behavior and psychological problems of young diabetic patients: A ten to twenty year survey. *Archives of Internal Medicine, 78*, 711–732.

Fitzelle, G. (1959). Personality factors and certain attitudes toward child rearing among parents of asthmatic children. *Psychosomatic Medicine, 21*, 208–217.

Fitzherbert, K. (1982). Communication with teachers in the health surveillance of school children. *Maternal and Child Health, 7*, 100–103.

Fölling, A. (1971). The original detection of phenylketonuria. In H. Bickel, F. P. Hudson, & L. I. Woolf (Eds.), *Phenylketonuria and some other inborn errors of amino acid metabolism* (pp. 1–17). Stuttgart: G. Thieme Verlag.

Francis, D. E. M. (1975). *Diets for sick children* (3rd ed.). Oxford: Blackwell Scientific.

Frankel, J. J. (1975). Juvenile diabetes—The look from within. In Z. Laron (Ed.), *Modern problems in paediatrics: Vol. 12. Diabetes in juveniles: Medical and rehabilitation aspects* (pp. 358–360). Basel: S. Kager.

Freeman, A. I., Wang, J. J., & Sinks, L. F. (1977). High-dose methotrexate in acute lymphocytic leukemia. *Cancer Treatment Reports, 61*, 727–731.

Freeman, E. H., Feingold, B. F., Schlesinger, K., & Gorman, F. J. (1964). Psychological variables in allergic disorders: A review. *Psychosomatic Medicine, 24*, 543–575.

Freeman, N. H. (1972). Process and product in children's drawing. *Perception, 1*, 123–140.

Freeman, R. D. (1968). Emotional reactions of handicapped children. In S. Chess & A. Thomas (Eds.), *Annual progress in child psychiatry and child development* (pp. 379–395). New York: Brunner/Mazel.

French, T. M. (1950). Emotional conflict and allergy. *International Archives of Applied Immunology, 1*, 28–40.

French, T. M., & Alexander, F. (1941). Psychogenic factors in bronchial allergy. *Psychosomatic Medicine, Monograph* 4.

Friedman, S. B., Chodoff, P., Mason, J. W., & Hamburg, D. A. (1963). Behavioural observations on parents anticipating the death of a child. *Pediatrics, 32*, 610–625.

Frish, M., Galatzer, A., & Laron, Z. (1977). Child–parent attitudes towards diabetes. In Z. Laron (Ed.), *Pediatrics and adolescent endocrinology: Vol. 3. Psychological aspects of balance in juveniles.* Basel: Karger.

Furchgott, E. (1963). Behavioral effects of iodizing radiations 1955–61. *Psychological Bulletin, 60*, 157–199.

Futterman, E. H., & Hoffman, I. (1973). Crisis and adaptation in families of fatally ill children. In E. J. Anthony & C. Koupernick (Eds.), *The child in his family: The impact of disease and death* (pp. 127–143). New York: Wiley.

Galatzer, A., Frish, M., & Laron, Z. (1977). Changes in self-concept and feelings toward diabetic adolescents. In Z. Laron (Ed.), *Pediatric adolescent endocrinology: Vol. 3. Psychological aspects of balance of diabetes in juveniles.* Basel: Karger.

Garner, A. M., & Thompson, C. W. (1974a). Factors in the management of juvenile diabetes. *Pediatric Psychology, 2*, 6–7.

Garner, A. M., & Thompson, C. W. (1974b). Juvenile diabetes. In P. R. Magreb (Ed.), *Psychological management of pediatric problems. Vol. I. Early life conditions and chronic diseases* (pp. 221–258). Baltimore: University Park Press.

Garner, A. M., Thompson, C. W., & Partridge, J. W. (1969). Who knows best? *Diabetes Bulletin, 45*, 3–4.

Garson, A., Benson, R. S., Ivler, L., & Patton, C. (1978). Parental reactions to children with congenital heart disease. *Child Psychiatry and Human Development, 9*(2), 86–94.

Gath, A. (1972). The mental health of siblings of congenitally abnormal children. *Journal of Child Psychology and Psychiatry, 13*, 211–218.

Gath, A. (1973). The school age sibling of mongol children. *British Journal of Psychiatry, 123*, 161–167.

Gath, A., Smith, M. A., & Baum, J. D. (1980). Emotional, behavioural and educational disorders in diabetic children. *Archives of Disease in Childhood, 55*, 371–375.

Gellert, E. (1958). Reducing the emotional stresses of hospitalization for children. *American Journal of Occupational Therapy, 12*, 125–129.

Gellert, E. (1961). *Children's beliefs about bodily illness.* Paper presented at the meeting of the American Psychological Association, New York.

Gellert, E. (1962). Children's conceptions of the content and functions of the human body. *Genetic Psychology Monographs, 65*, 293–411.

George, S. L., Fernbach, D. J., Vietti, T. J., Sullivan, M. P., Lane, D. M., Haggard, M. E., Berry, D. H., Lonsdale, D., & Komp, D. (1973). Factors influencing survival in pediatric acute leukemia. *The SWCCSG experience 1958–1970. Cancer, 32*, 1542–1553.

Gil, R., Frish, M., Amir, S., & Galatzer, A. (1977). Awareness of complications among juvenile diabetics and their parents. In Z. Laron (Ed.), *Pediatric adolescent endocrinology: Vol. 3: Psychological aspects of balance in juveniles.* Basel: Karger.

Gilmore, J. B. (1965). Play: A special behavior. In R. N. Haber (Ed.), *Current research in motivation* (pp. 343–355). New York: Holt, Rinehart & Winston.

Gochman, D. S. (1971). Children's perceptions of vulnerability to illness and accidents: A replication, extension and refinement. *HSMHA Health Service Report, 86,* 247–252.

Gochman, D. S., Bagramian, R. A., & Sheiham, A. (1972). Consistency in children's perceptions of vulnerability to health problems. *HSMHA Health Service Report, 87,* 282–288.

Goffman, H., Buckman, W., & Schade, G. H. (1957). The child's emotional response to hospitalization. *American Journal of Disease of Children, 93,* 157–164.

Goldberg, S. (1979). Premature birth: Consequences for the parent–infant relationship. *American Scientist, 67,* 214–220.

Goldberg, S., Brachfeld, S., & Divitto, B. (1980). Feeding, fussing and play: Parent infant interaction in the first year as a function of newborn status. In T. Field, S. Goldberg, D. Stern, & A. Sostek (Eds.), *Interactions of high risk infants and children* (pp. 133–153). New York: Academic Press.

Goldin, G. J., Perry, S. L., Margolin, R. J., Stotsky, B. A., & Foster, J. C. (1971). *The rehabilitation of the young epileptic.* Lexington, MA: Heath.

Goldstein, A., & Frankenburg, W. (1970). Behavioral consequences of dietary discontinuation in phenylketonuric children. Paper presented at *American Pediatric Society and Society for Pediatric Research,* Atlantic City, NJ, April, 29–May 2, p. 282.

Goldstein, L. (1980). *Relationship of health locus of control and individual diabetic management.* Unpublished master's thesis, Pace University, New York.

Goodall, J. (1976). Behaviour disorder: A preventable late sequel of illness in childhood. *Developmental Medicine and Child Neurology, 18,* 94–96.

Gordon, M., Crouthamel, C., Post, E. M., & Richman, R. A. (1982). Psychosocial aspects of constitutional short stature: Social competence, behavior problems, self-esteem, and family functioning. *Journal of Pediatrics, 101,* 477–480.

Goslin, E. R. (1978). Hospitalization as a life-crisis for the preschool child: A critical review. *Journal of Community Health, 3,* 321–356.

Goss, R. M. (1970). Language used by mothers of deaf children and mothers of hearing children. *American Annals of the Deaf, 115,* 93–96.

Gough, H. (1964). *The California psychological inventory manual* (rev. ed.). Palo Alto, CA. Consulting Psychologists Press.

Gough, H. (1975). *Manual for the California psychological inventory.* Palo Alto, CA: Consulting Psychologists Press.

Graham, P. J., Rutter, M. L., Yule, W., & Pless, I. B. (1967). Childhood asthma: A psychosomatic disorder? Some epidemiological considerations. *British Journal of Preventive and Social Medicine, 21,* 78–85.

Grave, G. D. (1974). The impact of chronic childhood illness on sibling development. In G. Grave & I. B. Pless (Eds.), *Fogarty International Center Series on the Teaching of Preventive Medicine: Vol. 3. Chronic childhood illness: Assessment of outcome* (pp. 225–232). (DHEW Publication No. NIH 76-877). Washington, DC: U.S. Government Printing Office.

Grave, G. D., & Pless, I. B. (Eds.) (1974). *Fogarty International Center Series on the Teaching of Preventive Medicine: Vol. 3. Chronic childhood illness: Assessment of outcome* (DHEW Publication No. NIH 76-877). Washington, DC: U.S. Government Printing Office.

Green, D. M., Freeman, A. I., & Sather, H. N. (1980). Comparison of three methods of central nervous system prophylaxis in childhood acute lympho-blastic leukaemia. *Lancet, 1*, 1398–1401.

Green, M., & Levitt, E. E. (1962). Constriction of body image in children with congenital heart disease. *Pediatrics, 29*, 438–441.

Greene, P. (1975). The child with leukemia in the classroom. *American Journal of Nursing, 75*, 86–87.

Greenfield, N. S. (1958). Allergy and the need for recognition. *Journal of Consulting Psychology, 22*, 230–232.

Gudmondsson, G. (1966). Epilepsy in Iceland: A clinical and epidemiological investigation. *Acta Neurologica Scandinavica*, (Suppl. 25), pp. 1–124.

Hackney, J. M., Hanley, W. B., Davidson, W., & Lindsao, L. (1968). Phenyl-ketonuria: Mental development, behavior and termination of low phenyl-alanine diet. *Journal of Pediatrics, 72*, 646–655.

Hamburg, D. A. (1974). Coping in life-threatening circumstances. *Psychotherapy and Psychosomatics, 23*, 13–25.

Hanley, W. B., Linsao, L., Davidson, W., & Moes, C. A. F. (1970). Malnutrition in early treatment of phenylketonuria. *Pediatric Research, 4*, 318–327.

Hardisty, R. M., & Till, M. M. (1968). Acute leukemia 1959–64. Factors affecting prognosis. *Archives of Disease in Childhood, 43*, 107–115.

Hardy, R. E. (1968). A study of manifest anxiety among blind residential school students. *New Outlook for the Blind, 48*, 173–175.

Harkavy, J., Johnson, S. B., Silverstein, J., Spillar, R., McCallum, M., & Rosenbloom, A. (1983). Who learns what at diabetes summer camp? *Journal of Pediatric Psychology, 8*, 143–153.

Harris, I. D., Rapaport, L., Rynerson, M. A., & Samter, M. (1950). Observations on asthmatic children. *American Journal of Orthopsychiatry, 20*, 490–505.

Heisel, J. S., Ream, S., & Raitz, R. (1973). The significance of life events as contributing factors in diseases of children. *Journal of Pediatrics, 83*, 119–123.

Heller, J. A. (1967). *The hospitalized child and his family*. Baltimore: John Hopkins Press.

Henggeler, S. W., & Cooper, P. F. (1983). Deaf child—hearing mother interaction: Extensiveness and reciprocity. *Journal of Pediatric Psychology, 8*, 83–96.

Hewett, S., Newson, J., & Newson, E. (1970). *The family and the handicapped child*. Chicago: Aldine.

Hill, R. (1965). Generic features of families under stress. In H. J. Parad (Ed.), *Crisis intervention: Selected readings* (pp. 32–52). New York: Family Service Association of America.

Holmes, H. A., & Holmes, F. F. (1975). After ten years, what are the handicaps and life-styles of children treated for cancer? An examination of the present status of 124 survivors. *Clinics in Pediatrics, 14*, 819–823.

Holmes, T. H.., & Rahe, R. H. (1967).The social readjustment rating scale. *Journal of Psychosomatic Research, 11*, 213–217.

Hoorweg, J., & Stanfeld, J. P. (1976). The effects of protein energy malnutrition in early childhood on intellectual and motor abilities in later childhood and adolescence. *Developmental Medicine and Child Neurology, 18*, 330–350.

Howarth, R. V. (1972). The psychiatry of terminal illness in children. *Proceedings of the Royal Society of Medicine, 65*, 1039–1040.

Hsia, D. Y. Y. (1967). Phenylketonuria. *Developmental Medicine and Child Neurology, 9*, 531–540.

Hsia, D. Y. Y., & Holtzman, N. A. (1973). A critical evaluation of PKU screening. In V. A. McKusick & R. Claiborne (Eds.), *Medical genetics*. New York: H. P. Publishing.

Hudson, F. P., Mordaunt, V. L., & Leahy, I. (1970). Evaluation of treatment begun in first three months of life in 184 cases of phenylketonuria. *Archives of Disease in Childhood, 45*, 5–12.

Hughes, J. (1976). The emotional impact of chronic disease: The pediatrician's responsibility. *American Journal of Diseases of Children, 130*, 1200–1203.

Hurt, C. H. (1976). Psychological and social aspects. In C. D. Boone (Ed.), *Comprehensive management of hemophilia*. Philadelphia: F. A. Davis.

Hurwitz, J., Kaplan, D. M., & Kaiser, E. (1962). Designing an instrument to assess parental coping mechanisms. *Social Casework, 10*, 527–532.

Hustu, H. O., & Aur, R. J. A. (1978). Extramedullary Leukaemia. *Clinics in Haematology, 7*, 313–337.

Iverson, T. (1966). Leukaemia in infancy and childhood. *Acta Paediatrica Scandinavica*, (Suppl. 167), pp. 1–219.

Ivey, J., Brewer, E. J., & Giannini, E. H. (1981). Psychosocial functioning in children with juvenile rheumatoid arthritis (JMA). *Arthritis and Rheumatism, 24*, S100.

Jackson, E. B. (1942). Treatment of the young child in the hospital. *American Journal of Orthopsychiatry, 12*, 56–62.

Janis, I. L. (1958). *Psychosocial stress*. New York: Wiley.

Jannoun, L. (1983). Are cognitive and educational development affected by age at which prophylactic therapy is given in acute leukeamia? *Archives of Disease in Childhood, 58*, 953–958.

Jay, S. M., Elliot, C. H., Ozdins, M., & Olson, R. (1984). *Behavioral management of distress in pediatric cancer patients undergoing painful medical procedures*. Manuscript submitted for publication.

Jay, S. M., Elliot, C. H., Ozolins, M., & Olson, R. (in press). Behavioral management of distress in pediatric cancer patients undergoing painful medical procedures. *Behavior, Research, and Therapy*.

Jennison, M. (1976). The pediatrician and care of chronic illness. *Pediatrics, 58*, 5–7.

Jessner, L., Blom, G. E., & Waldfogel, S. (1952). Emotional implications of tonsillectomy and adenoidectomy on children. *The Psychoanalytic Study of the Child, 7*, New York, International Universities Press.

Johnson, C. F. (1979). Phenylketonuria: A diagnosis that affects the entire family. *Medical Times, 107*, 37–40.

Johnson, C. N., & Wellman, H. M. (1982). Children's developing conceptions of the mind and brain. *Child Development, 53*, 222–234.

Johnson, S. B. (1980). Psychological factors in juvenile diabetes: A review. *Journal of Behavioral Medicine, 3*, 95–116.

Johnson, S. B., Pollak, T., Silverstein, J. H., Rosenbloom, A. L., Spillar, R., McCallum, M., & Harkavy, J. (1982). Cognitive and behavioral knowledge about insulin dependent diabetes among children and parents. *Pediatrics, 69,* 708–713.

Johnston, D., & Tattersall, R. (1981). Diabetes in childhood. In D. Hull (Ed.), *Recent advances in paediatrics* (pp. 195–212). London & Edinburgh: Churchill-Livingstone.

Jones, R. H. T., & Jones, R. S. (1966). Ventilatory capacity in young adults with a history of asthma in childhood. *British Medical Journal, 2,* 976–978.

Jones, R. S., Buston, M. H., & Wharton, M. J. (1962). The effect of exercise on ventilatory function in the child with asthma. *British Journal of Diseases of the Chest, 56,*78–86.

Kang, E. S., Kennedy, J. L., Gates, L., Burwash, I., & McKinnon, A. (1965). Clinical observations in PKU. *Pediatrics, 35,* 932–943.

Kang, E. S., Sallee, N. D., & Gerald, P. S. (1970). Results of treatment and termination of the diet in phenylketonuria. *Pediatrics, 46,* 881–890.

Kaplan, D. M., Grobstein, R., & Smith, A. (1976). Predicting the impact of severe illness in families. *Health and Social Work, 1,* 712–82.

Kaplan, D. M., Smith, A., Grobstein, R., & Fischman, S. E. (1973). Family mediation of stress. *Social Work, 18,* 60–69.

Kapotes, C. (1977). Emotional factors in chronic asthma. *Journal of Asthma Research, 5*(1), 5–14.

Katz, A. H. (1963). Social adaptation in chronic illness: A study of hemophilia. *American Journal of Public Health, 53,* 1666–1675.

Katz, E. R., Kellerman, J., Rigler, D., Williams, K. O., & Siegel, S. E. (1977). School intervention with pediatric cancer patients. *Journal of Pediatric Psychology, 2*(2), 72–76.

Katz, E. R., Kellerman, J., & Siegel, S. (1980). Behavioral distress in children undergoing medical procedures: Developmental considerations. *Journal of Consulting and Clinical Psychology, 49*(3), 470–471.

Katz, P. (1957). Behavior problems in juvenile diabetes. *Canadian Medical Association Journal, 76,* 738–743.

Kaufman, A. S. (1975). Factor analysis of the WISC-R at 11 age levels between 6½ and 16½ years. *Journal of Consulting and Clinical Psychology, 43,* 135–147.

Kaufman, A. S. (1976). Verbal-performance IQ discrepancies on the WISC-R. *Journal of Consulting and Clinical Psychology, 44,* 739–744.

Kaufman, R. V., & Hersher, B. (1971). Body-image changes in teenage diabetes. *Pediatrics, 48,* 123–128.

Keleske, L., Solomon, G., & Opitz, E. (1967). Parental reactions to phenylketonuria in the family. *Journal of Pediatrics, 70,* 793–798.

Keller, M. (1953). Progress in school of children in a sample of families in the eastern health district of Baltimore, Maryland. *Milbank Memorial Fund Quarterly, 31,* 391–410.

Kellerman, J. (Ed.) (1980). *Psychological aspects of childhood cancer.* Springfield, IL: C. C. Thomas.

Kellerman, J. (1983). Wishing doesn't make it so: A close look at Stehbens' "refutation." *Journal of Pediatric Psychology, 8*(4), 383–386.

Kellerman, J., Moss, H. A., & Siegel, S. E. (1982). WISC-R verbal performance discrepancy in children with cancer: A statistical quirk? *Journal of Pediatric Psychology, 7,* 263–266.

Kellock, T. D. (1970). Residential care of the diabetic chld. *Postgraduate Medical Journal, 46,* 629–630.

Kennedy, W. B. (1955). Psychological problems of the young diabetic. *Diabetes, 4,* 207–209.

Kessler, J. W. (1977). Parenting the handicapped child. *Pediatric Annals, 6,* 654–661.

Kister, M. C., & Patterson, C. J. (1980). Children's conceptions of the causes of illness: Understanding of contagion and use of immanent justice. *Child Development, 51,* 839–846.

Klaus, M. H., Kennell, J. H., Plumb, N., & Zuehlke, S. (1970). Human maternal behavior at the first contact with her young. *Pediatrics, 46,* 187–192.

Knox, W. E. (1960). An evaluation of treatment of phenylketonuria with diets low in phenylalanine. *Pediatrics, 26,* 1–11.

Koch, R., Dobson, J. C., Blaskovics, M., Williamson, M. C., Ernest, A. E., Friedman, E. G., & Parker, C. E. (1973). Collaborative study of children treated for phenylketonuria. In J. W. T. Seakins, R. A. Saunders, & C. Toothill (Eds.), *Treatent of inborn errors of metabolism* (pp. 3–18). Edinburgh & London: Churchill Livingstone.

Koff, E. , Boyle, P., & Pueschel, S. (1977). Perceptual–motor functioning in children with PKU. *American Journal of Diseases of Children, 13,* 1084–1087.

Kohrman, A. F., & Weil, W. B. (1971). Juvenile diabetes mellitus. *Advances in Pediatrics, 18,* 123–149.

Komrower, G. M. (1974). The philosophy and practice of screening for inherited diseases. *Pediatrics, 53,* 182–188.

Komrower, M., Saroharwalla, I. B., Coutts, J. M. J., & Ingham, D. (1979). Management of maternal phenylketonuria: An emerging clinical problem. *British Medical Journal, 1,* 1383–1387.

Koocher, G. P. (1981). Children's conceptions of death. In R. Bibace & M. E. Walsh (Eds.), *Children's conceptions of health, illness and bodily functions.* San Francisco: Jossey-Bass. pg. 85–99.

Koocher, G. P., & O'Malley, J. E. (1981). *The Damocles syndrome.* New York: McGraw-Hill.

Korsch, B. M., Negrette, V. F., Gardner, J. F., Weinstock, C. L., Mercer, A. S., Grushkin, C. M., & Fine, R. N. (1973). Kidney transplantation in children: Psychological follow-up study on child and family. *Journal of Pediatrics, 83,* 399–408.

Koski, M. L. (1969). The coping processes in childhood diabetes. *Acta Paediatrica Scandinavia,* 198 (Suppl.), 7–56.

Koski, M. L., & Kumento, A. (1975). Adolescent development and behavior: A psychosomatic follow-up of childhood diabetes. In Z. Laron (Ed.), *Modern problems in paediatrics: Vol. 12. Diabetes in juveniles: Medical and rehabilitation aspects* (pp. 348–353). Basel: Karger.

Kovacs, M. (1981). *The psychosocial sequelae of the diagnosis of juvenile diabetes on the parents of the youngsters.* Paper presented at the 5th International Beilinson Symposium on Psychosocial Aspects of Diabetes in Children and Adolescents, Herzliya-on-See, Israel.

Kraepelien, S. (1964). Prognosis of asthma in childhood with special reference to pulmonary function and the value of specific hyposensitisation. *Acta Paediatrica Scandinavica, 104*(Suppl.) 87–116.

Kübler-Ross, E. (1969). *On death and dying.* New York: Macmillan.

Kucia, C., Drotar, D., Doershuk, C. F., Stern, R. C., Boat, T. F., & Mathews, L. (1979). Home observation of family interaction and childhood adjustment to cystic fibrosis. *Journal of Pediatric Psychology, 4*(2), 189–195.

Kupst, M. J., Schulman, J. L., Honig, G., Maurer, H., Morgan, E., & Fochtman, D. (1982). Family coping with childhood leukaemia: One year after diagnosis. *Journal of Pediatric Psychology, 7,* 157–174.

Kuzemko, J. A. (Ed.). (1980). *Asthma in children.* Tunbridge Wells: Pitman Medical.

Lambert, C. N., Hamilton, R. C., & Pellicore, R. J. (1969). The juvenile amputee program: Its social and economic value. *Journal of Bone and Joint Surgery, 51-A,* 1135–1138.

Land, S., & Vineberg, S. E. (1965). Locus of control in blind children. *Exceptional children, 31,* 257–260.

Langdell, J. I. (1965). PKU: Eight year evaluation of treatment. *Archives of General Psychiatry, 12,* 363–367.

Langford, W. F. (1948). Physical illness and convalescence: Their meaning to the child. *Pediatrics, 33,* 242–250.

Lansdown, R. (1980). *More than sympathy: The everyday needs of sick and handicapped children.* London: Tavistock.

Laron, Z., Karp, M., & Frankel, J. J. (1972). *A study of the rehabilitation of juvenile and adolescent diabetics in the central region of Israel. Final Report.* Petach-Tiqva, Israel.

Laurendeau, M., & Pinard, A. (1962). *Causal thinking in the child.* (pp. 11–13). New York: International Universities Press.

Laurendeau, M., & Pinard, A. (1970). *Development of the concept of space in the child.* New York: International Universities Press.

Lavigne, J. V., & Burns, W. J. (1981). *Pediatric psychology: Introduction for pediatricians and psychologists.* New York: Grune & Stratton.

Lavigne, J . V., & Ryan, M. (1979). Psychological adjustment of siblings of children with chronic illness. *Pediatrics, 63,* 616–627.

Lazarus, R. S. (1966). *Psychological stress and the coping process.* New York: McGraw-Hill.

Lefcourt, H. M. (1972). Recent developments in the study of locus of control. In B. A. Maher (Ed.), *Progress in experimental personality research: Vol. 6* (pp. 1–39). New York: Academic Press.

Leifer, A. D., Leiderman, P. H., Barnett, C. R., & Williams, J. A. (1972). Effects of mother–infant separation on maternal attachment behavior. *Child Development, 43,* 1203–1218.

Leigh, D., & Marley, E. (1956). A psychiatric assessment of adult asthmatics: A statistical study. *Journal of Psychosomatic Research, 1,* 128–136.

Leonard, C. O., Chase, G. A., & Childs, B. (1972). Genetic counselling: A consumer's view. *New England Journal of Medicine, 287,* 433–439.

Levenson, P. M., Copeland, D. R., Morrow, J. R., Pfefferbaum, B., & Silberberg, Y. (1983). Disparities in disease-related perceptions of adolescent cancer patients and their parents. *Journal of Pediatric Psychology, 8*(1), 33–45.

Leveque, B., Jean, R., Benoit, M. R., Cloup, I., Mischler, J., & Marie, J. (1969). Evolution, prognostic éloigné et retenissement social de la maladie asthmatique de l'enfant. *Annales de Pediatrie, 45*, 1459–1463.

Levy, E. (1959). Children's behavior under stress and its relation to training by parents to respond to stress functions. *Child Development, 30*, 307–324.

Lewis, B. L., & Khaw, K. T. (1982). Family functioning as a mediating variable affecting psychosocial adjustment of children with cystic fibrosis. *Journal of Pediatrics, 101*(4), 636–640.

Lewis, I. C. (1967). Leukaemia in childhood: Its effects on the family. *Australian Paediatric Journal, 3*, 244–247.

Ley, P. (1982). Giving information to patients. In J. R. Eiser (Ed.), *Social psychology and behavioral medicine* (pp. 339–374). Chichester: John Wiley & Sons.

Li, F., & Stone, R. (1976). Survivors of cancer in childhood. *Annals of Internal Medicine, 84*, 551–553.

Light, P. (1983). Social interaction and cognitive development: A review of post-Piagetian research. In S. Meadows (Ed.), *Developing thinking: Approaches to children's cognitive development* (pp. 67–88). London: Methuen.

Lilienfeld, A. M., & Parkhurst, E. (1951). A study of the association of factors of pregnancy and parturition with the development of cerebral palsy: A preliminary report. *American Journal of Hygiene, 53*, 262–282.

Linde, L. M., Rosof, B., Dunn, O. J., & Rabb, E. (1966). Attitudinal factors in congenital heart disease. *Pediatrics, 38*, 92–101.

Lindemann, J. E. (Ed.) (1981). *Psychological and behavioral aspects of physical disability*. New York: Plenum Press.

Lindsay, J., Ounsted, C., & Richards, P. (1979). Long-term outcome in children with temporal lobe seizures. Social outcome and childhood factors. *Developmental Medicine and Child Neurology, 21*, 285–298.

Lipowski, Z. J. (1970). Physical illness, the individual and the coping process. *Psychiatry in Medicine, 1*, 91–98.

Lipsett, L. P. (1958). A self-concept scale for children and its relationship to the children's form of the Manifest Anxiety Scale. *Child Development, 29*, 463–472.

Little, S. W., & Cohen, L. D. (1951). Goal-setting behavior of asthmatic children and of their mothers for them. *Journal of Personality, 19*, 376–389.

Long, R. T., Lamont, J. E., Whipple, B., Bandler, L., Blom, G. E., Burgin, L., & Jessner, L. (1958). A psychosomatic study of allergic and emotional factors in children with asthma. *American Journal of Psychiatry, 114*(10), 890–899.

Lowe, T. L., Tanaka, K., Seashore, M. R., Young, G. J., & Cohen, D. (1980). Detection of phenylketonuria in autistic and psychotic children. *Journal of the American Medical Association, 243*, 126–128.

Lowery, B. J., & Ducette, J. P. (1976). Disease-related learning and disease control in diabetes as a function of locus of control. *Nursing Research, 25*, 358–362.

Lucas, O. N. (1965). Dental extractions in the hemophiliac: Control of emotional factors by hypnosis. *American Journal of Clinical Hypnosis, 7*, 301–307.

Lynn, D. B., Glaser, H. H., & Harrison, G. S. (1962). Comprehensive medical care for handicapped children: III concepts of illness in children with rheumatic fever. *American Journal of Diseases of Children, CIII* (February), 42–50.

MacCarthy, M. (1975). Social aspects of treatment in childhood leukaemia. *Social Science and Medicine, 9*, 263–269.

Maddison, D., & Raphael, B. (1971). Social and psychological consequences of chronic disease in childhood. *Medical Journal of Australia, 2*, 1265–1270.

Madge, N. (Ed.). (1972). *Families at risk*. London: Heinemann Educational Books.

Maguire, G. P. (1983). Psychological and social aspects of childhood malignancy. *Annals Nestlé, 41*(2), 32–43.

Maguire, P., Comaroff, J., Ramsell, P. J., & Morris-Jones, P. H. (1979). Psychological and social problems in families of children with leukaemia. In P. H. Morris-Jones (Ed.), *Topics in paediatrics: Vol. 1. Haematology and oncology* (pp. 141–149). London: Pitman Medical.

Mahaffy, P. (1965). The effects of hospitalization on children admitted for tonsillectomy and adenoidectomy. *Nursing Research, 14*, 12–19.

Malone, J., Hellrung, I., Malphus, E., Rosenbloom, A. L., Grgic, M. D., & Weber, F. T. (1976). Good diabetic control: A study in mass delusion. *Journal of Pediatrics, 88*, 943–947.

Markova, I., Stirling-Phillips, J., & Forbes, C. D. (1984). The use of tools by children with haemophilia. *Journal of Child Psychology and Psychiatry and Allied Disciplines, 25*, 261–272.

Martin, A. J., Landau, L. I., & Phelan, P. D. (1982). Asthma from childhood at age 21: The patient and his disease. *British Medical Journal, 284*, 380–382.

Mattson, A. (1972). Long-term physical illness in childhood: A challenge to psychosocial adaptation. *Pediatrics, 50*, 801–811.

Mattson, A. (1975). Psychological aspects of childhood asthma. *Pediatric Clinics of North America, 2211*, 77–88.

Mattson, A., & Gross, S. (1966). Adaptational and defensive behavior in young hemophiliacs and their parents. *American Journal of Psychiatry, 122*, 1349–1356.

Mattson, A., Gross, S., & Hall, T. W. (1971). Psychoendocrine study of adaptation in young hemophiliacs. *Psychosomatic Medicine, 33*, 215–225.

Matus, I., Kinsman, R. A., & Jones, N. F. (1978). Pediatric patient attitudes toward chronic asthma and hospitalization. *Journal of Chronic Diseases, 31*, 611–618.

McAnarney, E., Pless, I. B., Satterwhite, B., & Friedman, S. (1974). Psychological problems of children with chronic juvenile arthritis. *Pediatrics, 53*, 523–528.

McBean, M. S., & Stephenson, J. B. (1968). Treatment of classical phenylketonuria. *Archives of Disease in Childhood, 43*, 1–7.

McCarthy, D. (1970). *McCarthy scales of children's abilities*. New York: Psychological Corporation.

McCollum, A. T. (1981). *The chronically ill child: A guide for parents and professionals*. New Haven, CT: Yale University Press.

McCollum, A. T., & Gibson, L. E. (1970). Family adaptation to the child with cystic fibrosis. *Journal of Pediatrics, 77*, 517–578.

McCormick, M. C., Shapiro, S., & Starfield, B. (1982). Factors associated with maternal opinion of infant development—Clues to the vulnerable child? *Pediatrics, 69*(5), 537–543.

McCraw, R., & Tuma, J. (1977). Rorschach content categories of juvenile diabetics. *Psychological Reports, 40*, 818–821.

McCue, K. (1980). Preparing children for medical procedures. In J. Kellerman (Ed.), *Psychological aspects of childhood cancer*. Springfield, IL: C. C. Thomas.

McFie, J., & Robertson, J. (1973). Psychological test results of children with thalidomide disorders. *Developmental Medicine and Child Neurology, 15*, 719–727.

McGavin, A. P., Schultz, E., Peden, G. W., & Bowen, B. D. (1940). The physical growth, the degree of intelligence and the personality adjustment of a group of diabetic children. *New England Journal of Medicine, 223*, 119–124.

McLean, J., & Ching, A. (1973). Follow-up study of relationships between family situation and bronchial asthma in children. *Journal of American Academy of Child Psychiatry, 12*, 142–161.

McMichael, J. (1971). *Handicap: A study of physically handicapped children and their families*. Pittsburg: University of Pittsburg Press.

McNemar, Q. (1962). *Psychological statistics*. New York and London: Wiley.

Meadow, K. P. (1975). The development of deaf children. In E. M. Hetherington (Ed.), *Review of child development research: Vol. 5* (pp. 441–508). Chicago: University of Chicago Press.

Meadows, A. T., Massari, D. J., Ferguson, J., Gordon, J., Littman, P., & Moss, K. (1981). Declines in IQ scores and cognitive dysfunctions in children with acute lympocytic leukaemia treated with cranial irradiation. *Lancet, 2*, 1015–1018.

Mechanic, D. (1964). The influence of mothers on their children's health attitudes and behavior. *Pediatrics, 33*, 444–453.

Mechanic, D. (1968). *Medical sociology—A selective view*. New York: Free Press.

Mechanic, D. (1979). The stability of health and illness behavior: Results from a 16-year follow-up. *American Journal of Public Health, 69*, 1142–1145.

Medical Research Council Working Party (1968). Present status of different mass screening procedures for phenylketonuria. *British Medical Journal, 4*, 7–13.

Medical Research Council (1973). Treatment of acute lymphoblastic leukaemia: Effect of 'prophylactic' therapy against central nervous system leukaemia. *British Medical Journal, 2*, 381–384.

Medical Research Council (1978). Effects of varying radiation schedule, cyclophosamide treatment and duration of treatment in acute lymphoblastic leukaemia. *British Medical Journal, 2*, 787–791.

Melamed, B. C., Meyer, R., Gee, C., & Soule, L. (1976). The influence of time and type of hospitalization. *Journal of Pediatric Psychology, 5*, 31–37.

Melamed, B. C., & Siegel, L. J. (1975). Reduction of anxiety in children facing hospitalization and surgery by use of filmed modeling. *Journal of Consulting and Clinical Psychology, 43,* 511–521.

Mellish, R. W. (1969). Preparation of a child for hospitalization and surgery. *Pediatric Clinics of North America, 16,* 543–553.

Melnick, C. R., Michaels, K. K., & Matalon, R. (1981). Linguistic development of children with phenylketonuria and normal intelligence. *Journal of Pediatrics, 98,* 269–272.

Menolascino, F. J., & Egger, M. L. (1978). *Medical dimensions of mental retardation.* Lincoln, NE: University of Nebraska Press.

Meyer, R. J., & Haggerty, R. J. (1962). Streptococcal infections in families: Factors altering individual susceptibility. *Pediatrics, 29,* 539–549.

Meyerowitz, J. H., & Kaplan, H. B. (1967). Familial responses to stress: The care of cystic fibrosis. *Social Science and Medicine, 1,* 249–266.

Miller, H., & Baruch, D. W. (1948). Psychosomatic studies of children with allergic manifestations. 1. Maternal rejection: A study of 63 cases. *Psychosomatic Medicine, 10,* 275–278.

Miller, H., & Baruch, D. W. (1967). The emotional problems of childhood and their relation to asthma. In I. Frank & M. Powell (Eds.), *Psychomatic ailments in childhood and adolescence.* Springfield, IL: C. C. Thomas.

Miller, J. J., Spitz, P. W., Simpson, V., & Williams, G. F. (1982). The social function of young adults who had arthritis in childhood. *Journal of Pediatrics, 100,* 3, 378–382.

Millstein, S. G., Adler, N. E., & Irwin, C. E. (1981). Conceptions of illness in young adolescents. *Pediatrics, 68,* 834–839.

Minuchin, S., Baker, L., Rosman, B., Leibman, R., Milman, L., & Todd, T. (1975). A conceptual model of psychosomatic illness in children. *Archives of General Psychiatry, 32,* 1031–1038.

Miranda, P. M., & Horwitz, D. L. (1978). High fibre diets in the treatment of diabetes mellitus. *Annals of Internal Medicine, 88,* 482–486.

Mishler, E. G., Amarasingham, L. R., Hauser, S. T., Liem, R., Osherson, D. S., & Waxler, N. E. (1981). *Social contexts of health, illness and patient care* Cambridge, England: Cambridge University Press.

Mitchell, A. J., Frost, L., & Marx, J. R. (1953). Emotional aspects of pediatric allergy—The role of the mother–child relationship. *Annals of Allergy, 11,* 744–751.

Mitchell, R. G., & Dawson, B. (1973). Educational and social characteristics of children with asthma. *Archives of Disease in Childhood, 48,* 467–471.

Moen, J. L., Wilcox, R. D., & Burns, J. K. (1977). PKU as a factor in the development of self-esteem. *Behavioral Pediatrics, 90,* 1027–1029.

Moffatt, M. E. K., & Pless, I. B. (1983). Locus of control in juvenile diabetic campers: Changes during camp, and relationship to camp staff assessments. *Journal of Pediatrics, 103,* 146–150.

Moos, R., & Moos, B. (1976). A typology of family social environments. *Family Process, 15,* 357–372.

Moos, R. H., & Tsu, V. D. (1977). The crisis of physical illness: An overview. In R. H. Moos (Ed.), *Coping with physical illness.* New York: Plenum Press.

Morris, R. P. (1959). Effect of the mother on goal setting behavior of the asthmatic child. *Dissertation Abstracts, 20,* 1440.

Morrissey, J. R. (1964). Death anxiety in children with a fatal illness. *American Journal of Psychotherapy, 8*, 606–615.

Morrison-Smith, J., Harding, L. K., & Cumming, G. (1971). The changing prevalence of asthma in school children. *Clinical Allergy, 1*, 57–61.

Moss, H. A., Nannis, E. D., & Poplack, D. G. (1981). The effects of prophylactic treatment of the central nervous system on the intellectual functioning of children with acute lymphocytic leukemia. *American Journal of Medicine, 71*, 47–52.

Mugny, G., Perret-Clermont, A. N., & Doise, W. (1981). Interpersonal co-ordinations and sociological differences in the construction of the intellect. In G. M. Stephenson & J. H. Davis (Eds.), *Progress in applied social psychology: Vol. 1* (pp. 315–343). Chichester, England: Wiley.

Mulhern, R. K., Crisco, J. J., & Camitta, B. M. (1981). Patterns of communication among pediatric patients with leukemia, parents, and physicians: Prognostic disagreements and misunderstandings. *Journal of Pediatrics, 99*, 480–483.

Myers-Vando, R., Steward, M. S., Folkins, C. H., & Hines, P. A. (1979). The effects of congenital heart disease on cognitive development, illness, causality concepts and vulnerability. *American Journal of Orthopsychiatry, 49*(4), 617–625.

Nagler, M. (1978). Psychological adjustment of long-term survivors of childhood cancer. *Dissertation Abstracts International, 39*, 1964-B.

Natapoff, J. (1978). Children's views of health. *American Journal of Public Health, 68*, 995–1000.

Natterson, J. M., & Knudson, A. G. (1960). Observations concerning fear of death in fatally ill children and their mothers. *Psychosomatic Medicine, 22*, 456–465.

Neligan, G. A., & Prudham, O. (1974). Family factors affecting child development. *Archives of Disease in Childhood, 51*, 853–858.

Nesbit, M. E., Sather, H. N., & Robinson, L. (1981). Presymptomatic central nervous system therapy in previously untreated childhood acute lymphoblastic leukemia: Comparison of 1800rad and 2400rad. *Lancet, i*, 461–466.

Neuhaus, E. C. (1958). A personality study of asthmatic and cardiac children. *Psychosomatic Medicine, 20*, 181–186.

Neuhauser, C., Amsterdam, B., Hines, P., & Steward, M. (1978). Children's concepts of healing: Cognitive development and locus of control factors. *American Journal of Orthopsychiatry, 48*, 334–341.

Nowicki, S., & Strickland, B. R. (1973). A locus of control scale for children. *Journal of Consulting and Clinical Psychology, 40*, 148–154.

Nuffield Foundation (1963). *Children in hospital: Studies in planning.* New York: Oxford University Press.

Nuttall, F. Q. (1983). Diet and the diabetic patient. *Diabetes Care, 6*, 197–206.

Obetz, S. W., Smithson, W. A., & Groover, R. V. (1979). Neuropsychologic follow-up study of children with acute lymphocytic leukemia. *American Journal of Hematology and Oncology, 1*, 207–213.

Oliff, A., Bercu, B., & Dichiro, G. (1979). Abnormally low growth hormone responses to insulin induced hypoglycemia following central nervous system prophylaxis: Correlation with abnormal computerized tomographic brain scans. *Proceedings of the American Association of Cancer Research—American Society of Clinical Oncology, 20*, 393–397.

Oliver, L. I. (1977). The association of health attitudes and perceptions of youths 12–17 years of age with those of their parents. In *Vital and Health Statistics* (National Center for Health Statistics Series 11, No. 161, DHEW Publication HRA 77-1643). Washington, DC: U.S. Government Printing Office.

O'Malley, J. E., Koocher, G., Foster, D., & Slavin, L. (1979). Psychiatric sequelae of surviving childhood cancer. *American Journal of Orthopsychiatry, 49*, 608–616.

Orr, D. P., Weller, S. C., Satterwhite, B., & Pless, I. B. (1984). Psychosocial implications of chronic illness in adolescence. *Journal of Pediatrics, 104*, 152–157.

Palm, C. R., Murcek, M. A., Roberts, T. R., Mansmann, H. C., & Fireman, P. (1970). A review of asthma admissions and deaths at the children's Hospital of Pittsburg from 1935 to 1968. *Journal of Allergy, 46*, 257–269.

Palmer, B. B., & Lewis, C. E. (1975, October). *Development of health attitudes and behaviors*. Paper presented at the meeting of the American School Health Association, Denver.

Parcel, G. S., & Meyer, M. P. (1978). Development of an instrument to measure children's health locus of control. *Health Education Monographs, 6*, 149–159.

Parker, C. E. (1973). Remarks on the long-term aspects of phenylketonuria. In J. Seakins, R. Saunders, & C. Toothill (Eds.), *Treatment of inborn errors of metabolism* (pp. 19–21). Edinburgh & London: Churchill Livingstone.

Partridge, J. W., Garner, A. M., Thompson, C. W., & Cherry, T. (1972). Attitudes of adolescents toward their diabetes. *American Journal of Diseases of Children, 124*, 226–229.

Pasamanick, B., & Knobloch, H. (1961). Epidemiological studies on the complications of pregnancy and the birth process. In G. Caplan (Ed.), *Prevention of mental disorders in children* (pp. 74–94). New York: Basic Books.

Patterson, P. R., Denning, C., & Kutscher, A. H. (1973). *Psychological aspects of cystic fibrosis: A model for chronic lung disease*. New York: Columbia University.

Paulsen, E. P., & Colle, E. (1969). Diabetes Mellitus. In L. E. Garner (Ed.), *Endocrine and genetic diseases of childhood* (pp. 808–823). Philadelphia: W. B. Saunders.

Payne, J. S., Goff, J. R., & Paulson, M. A. (1980). Psychosocial adjustment of families following the death of a child. In J. L. Schulman & M. J. Kupst (Eds.), *The child with cancer* (pp. 183–193). Springfield, IL: C. C. Thomas.

Pearson, G. H. (1941). Effect of operative procedures on the emotional life of the child. *American Journal of Disease of Children, 62*, 716–729.

Pearson, J., & Dudley, H. A. F. (1982). Bodily perceptions in surgical patients. *British Medical Journal, 284*, 1545–1546.

Peck, B. (1979). Effects of childhood cancer on long-term survivors and their families. *British Medical Journal, 1*, 1327–1329.

Peckham, C., & Butler, R. (1978). A national study of asthma in childhood. *Journal of Epidemiology and Community Health, 32*, 79–85.

Pendleton, D., & Hasler, J. (Eds.) (1983). *Doctor–patient communication*. London: Academic Press.

Perret-Clermont, A. N. (1980). *Social interactions and cognitive development in children*. London: Academic Press.

Perrin, E. C., & Gerrity, P. S. (1979, May). *The development of concepts regarding illness*. Paper presented at the 19th Annual Meeting of the Ambulatory Pediatric Association, Atlanta.

Perrin, E. C., & Gerrity, P. S. (1981). There's a demon in your belly: Children's understanding of illness. *Pediatrics, 67*, 841–849.

Peshkin, M. (1968). Analysis of the role of residential asthma centers for children with intractable asthma. *Journal of Asthma Research, 6*(2), 59–92.

Peters, B. M. (1978). School-aged children's beliefs about causality of illness: A review of the literature. *Maternal–Child Nursing Journal, 7*(3), 143–155.

Peterson, L., & Ridley-Johnson, R. (1980). Pediatric hospital response to survey of prehospital preparation for children. *Journal of Pediatric Psychology, 5*, 1–7.

Peterson, L., & Shigetomi, C. (1983). One-year follow-up of elective surgery child patients receiving preoperative preparation. *Journal of Pediatric Psychology, 7*(1), 43–48.

Peylan-Ramu, N., Poplack, D. G., & Pizzo, P. A. (1978). Abnormal CT scans of the brain in asymptomatic children with acute lymphocytic leukemia after prophylactic treatment of the central nervous system with radiation and intrathecal chemotherapy. *New England Journal of Medicine, 298*, 815–818.

Piaget, J. (1930). *The child's conception of physical causality*. London: Routledge and Kegan Paul.

Piaget, J. (1962). *Play, dreams and imitation in childhood*. New York: W. W. Norton.

Piaget, J. (1962). The relation of affectivity to intelligence in the mental development of the child. *Bulletin of the Meninger Clinic, 26*, 129–137.

Piaget, J. (1970). Piaget's theory in P. H. Mussen (Ed.), *Carmichael's Manual of Child Psychiatry, Vol. 1*. New York: Wiley.

Piaget, J., & Inhelder, B. (1956). *The child's conception of space*. London, Routledge & Kegan Paul.

Piers, E. V., & Harris, D. B. (1964). Age and other correlates of self-concept in children. *Journal of Educational Psychology, 55*, 91–96.

Piness, G., Miller, H., & Sullivan, E. B. (1937). The intelligence rating of the allergic child. *Journal of Allergy, 8*, 168–174.

Pinkerton, P. (1974). Psychological problems of children with chronic illness. In (Ed.), *The care of children with chronic illness* (pp. 43–49). *Proceedings of 67th Conference on Pediatric Research*. Columbia, OH: Ross Laboratories.

Platt Committee, Great Britain (1959). *The welfare of children in hospitals*. London: Her Majesty's Stationery Office.

Pless, I. B., & Douglas, J. W. B. (1971). Chronic illness in childhood. 1. Epidemiological and clinical observations. *Pediatrics, 47*, 405–414.

Pless, I. B., & Pinkerton, P. (1975). *Chronic childhood disorder, Promoting patterns of adjustment*. London: Henry Kimpton.

Pless, I. B., & Roghmann, K. J. (1971). Chronic illness and its consequences:

Observations based on three epidemiological surveys. *Journal of Pediatrics, 79*, 351–359.

Pless, I. B., Roghmann, K. J., & Haggerty, R. J. (1972). Chronic illness, family functioning, psychological adjustment: A model for the allocation of preventive mental health services. *International Journal of Epidemiology, 1*, 271–277.

Pless, I. B., & Satterwhite, B. (1975). Chronic Illness. In R. J. Haggerty, K. J. Roghmann, & Pless, I. B. (Eds.), *Child health and the community*. New York: Wiley.

Pless, I., Satterwhite, B., & Van Vechten, D. (1976). Chronic illness in childhood: A regional survey of care. *Pediatrics, 58*, 37–46.

Porter, C. (1974). Grade school children's perceptions of their internal body parts. *Nursing Research, 23*, 384–391.

Powazek, M., Schyving Payne, J., Goff, J. R., Paulson, M. A., & Stagner, S. (1980). Psychosocial ramifications of childhood leukaemia: One year post-diagnosis. In J. L. Schulman & M. J. Kupst (Eds.), *The child with cancer: Clinical approaches to psychosocial care—Research in psychosocial aspects* (pp. 143–155). Springfield, IL: C. C. Thomas.

Pratt, L. (1973). Child rearing methods and children's health behaviors. *Journal of Health and Social Behavior, 14*, 61–69.

Price, R. A., & Jamieson, P. A. (1975). The central nervous system in childhood leukemia. II Subacute leukoencephalopathy. *Cancer, 35*, 306–318.

Prugh, D., Staub, E. M., Sands, H. H., Kirschbaum, R. M., & Lenihan, E. A. (1953). A study of the emotional reactions of children and families to hospitalization and illness. *American Journal of Orthopsychiatry, 23*, 70–106.

Pueschel, S. M., Yeatman, S., & Hum, C. (1977). Discontinuing the phenyl-alanine restricted diet in young children with phenylketonuria: Psychosocial aspects. *Journal of American Dietetics Association, 70*, 506–509.

Quinton, D., & Rutter, M. (1976). Early hospital admissions and later disturbances of behavior: An attempted replication of Douglas findings. *Developmental Medicine and Child Neurology, 18*, 447–459.

Rackemann, F. H., & Edwards, M. L. (1952). Asthma in childhood. Follow-up study of 688 patients after intervals of 20 years. *New England Journal of Medicine, 246*, 815–858.

Rachman, S., & Phillips, C. (1975). *Psychology and medicine*. London: Temple Smith.

Rainer, J. D., Altschuler, K. Z., & Kallman, F. J. (1963). *Family and mental health problems of a deaf population*. New York: Columbia University Press.

Rashkis, S. (1965). Child's understanding of health. *Archives of General Psychiatry, 12*, 10–17.

Rawls, D. J., Rawls, J. R., & Harrison, C. W. (1971). An investigation of six- to eleven-year-old children with allergic disorders. *Journal of Consulting and Clinical Psychology, 36*, 260–264.

Rhyne, M B. (1974). Incidence of atopic disease. *Medical Clinics of North America, 58*, 5–8.

Richardson, S. A., Hastorf, A. H., & Dornbusch, S. M. (1964). Effects of physical disability on a child's description of himself. *Child Development, 35*, 893–907.

Richman, N., & Graham, P. J. (1971). A behavioral screening questionnaire for use with three-year-old children. Preliminary findings. *Journal of Child Psychology and Psychiatry and Allied Disciplines, 12*, 5–33.

Richter, H. (1943). Emotional disturbances of constant pattern following nonspecific respiratory infection. *Journal of Pediatrics, 23*, 315–325.

Robertson, J. (1952). *A two-year-old goes to hospital* [Film]. New York: New York University Film Library.

Robertson, J. (1958a). *Going to hospital with mother* [Film]. New York: New York University Film Library.

Robertson, J. (1958b). *Young children in hospitals*. New York: Basic Books.

Robins, L. N., Bates, W. M., & O'Neil, P. (1962). Adult drinking patterns of former problem children. In D. Pittman & C. Snider (Eds.), *Society, culture and drinking patterns*. New York: Wiley.

Robinson, G. (1972). The story of parentectomy. *Journal of Asthma Research, 9*(4), 199–205.

Rodda, M. (1970). *The hearing imparied school leaver*. London: University of London Press.

Roghmann, K. J., & Haggerty, R. J. (1970). Rochester child health surveys. I. Objectives, organization and methods. *Medical Care, 8*, 47–54.

Rolle-Daya, H., Pueschel, S., & Lombroso, C. (1975). Electroencephalographic findings in children with phenylketonuria. *American Journal of Diseases of Children, 129*, 896–900.

Roskies, E. (1972). *Abnormality and normality: The mothering of thalidomide children*. Ithaca, NY: Cornell University Press.

Rotter, J. B. (1975). Some problems and misconceptions related to the construct of internal versus external control of reinforcement. *Journal of Consulting and Clinical Psychology, 43*, 56–67.

Rutter, M. (1967). A children's behavior questionnaire for completion by teachers: Preliminary findings. *Journal of Child Psychology and Psychiatry and Allied Disciplines, 8*, 1–12.

Rutter, M. (1975). *Helping troubled children*. London: Penguin.

Rutter, M. (1977). Brain damage syndromes in childhood: Concepts and findings. *Journal of Child Psychology and Psychiatry and Allied Disciplines, 18*, 1–22.

Rutter, M. (1981). Stress, coping and development: Some issues and some questions. *Journal of Child Psychology and Psychiatry and Allied Disciplines, 22*, 4, 323–356.

Rutter, M., Graham, P., & Yule, W. (1970). *Clinics in developmental medicine. No. 35/36. A Neuropsychiatric study in childhood*. London: SIMP/Heinemann.

Rutter, M., Quinton, D., Rowlands, O., Yule, W., & Berger, M. (1975). Attainment and adjustment in two geographical areas. III. Some factors accounting for area differences. *British Journal of Psychiatry, 126*, 520–528.

Rutter, M., Tizard, J., & Whitmore, K. (1970). *Education, health and behaviour*. London: Longman.

Rutter, M., Yule, B., Quinton, D., Rowlands, O., Yule, W., & Berger, M. (1975). Attainment and adjustment in two geographical areas. III Some Factors accounting for area differences. *British Journal of Psychiatry, 126*, 520–533.

Sadler, J. (1975). The long-term hospitalization of asthmatic children. *Pediatric Clinics of North America, 22*(1), 173–183.

St. James-Roberts, I. (1979). Neurological plasticity, recovery from brain insult and child development. In H. W. Reese & L. P. Lipsett (Eds.), *Advances in child psychology: Vol. 14* (pp. 254–315). New York: Academic Press.

Sameroff, A. J., & Chandler, M. J. (1975). Reproductive risk and the continuum of caretaking casualty. In F. D. Horowitz (Ed.), *Review of child development research* (pp. 187–243). Chicago: University of Chicago Press.

Sargent, J. (1982). Family systems theory and chronic childhood illness: Diabetes mellitus. In K. Flomenhaft & A. E. Christ (Eds.), *Psychosocial family interventions in chronic pediatric illness* (pp. 125–138). New York: Plenum Press.

Saugstad, L. F. (1972). Birth weights in children with phenylketonuria and their siblings. *Lancet 1*, 809–813.

Saul, L. J., & Lyons, J. W. (1951). The psychodynamics of respiration. In H. A. Abramson (Ed.), *Somatic and psychiatric treatment of asthma* (pp.93–103). Baltimore: Williams & Wilkins.

Sayed, A. J., & Leaverton, D. R. (1974). Kinetic-family drawings of children with diabetes. *Child Psychiatry and Human Development, 5*(1), 40–50.

Schafer, L. C., Glasgow, R. E., McCaul, K. D., & Dreher, M. (1983). Adherence to IDDM regimes: Relationship to psychosocial variables and metabolic control. *Diabetes Care, 6*, 493–498.

Schaffer, H. R., & Callendar, W. W. (1959). Psychological effects of hospitalization in infancy. *Pediatrics, 245*, 528–539.

Schecter, M. D. (1961). The orthopedically handicapped child. *Archives of General Psychiatry, 4* (March) 247–253.

Schild, S. (1979). Psychological issues in genetic counseling of PKU. In S. Kessler (Ed.), *Genetic counseling: Psychological dimensions* (pp. 135–152). New York: Academic Press.

Schilder, P., & Wechsler, D. (1935). What do children know about the interior of the body? *International Journal of Psychoanalysis, 16*, 345–350.

Schlesinger, H. S., & Meadow, K. P. (1972). *Sound and sign: Childhood deafness and mental health.* Berkeley: University of California Press.

Schmid-Rüter, E., & Grubel-Kaiser, S. (1977). Phenylketonuria: Fruherfassung und geistige Entwicklung. *Monatsschrift fur Kinderheilkunde, 125*, 479–481.

Schulman, J. (1976). *Coping with tragedy: Successfully facing the problem of a seriously ill child.* Chicago: Follett Publishing.

Schulman, J. L., & Kupst, M. J. (Eds.), (1980). *The child with cancer. Clinical approaches to psychosocial care: Research in psychosocial aspects.* Springfield, IL: C. C. Thomas.

Schuster, F. B. (1951). Pediatrics, social work and psychiatry overlapping disciplines. *Pediatrics, 7*, 449–452.

Schwartz, D. D. S., Albino, J. E., & Tedesco, L. (1983). Effects of psychological preparation on children hospitalized for dental operations. *Journal of Pediatrics, 102*, 634–638.

Seidel, V. P., Chadwick, O., & Rutter, M. (1975). Psychological disorders in crippled children: A comparative study of children with and without brain damage. *Developmental Medicine and Child Neurology, 17*, 553–563.

Seligman, M. E. P. (1975). *Helplessness.* San Francisco: Freeman.

Shaffer, D., Chadwick, O., & Rutter, M. (1975). Psychiatric outcome of localised head injury in children. In R. Porter & D. W. FitzSimons (Eds.), *CIBA Foundation Symposium No. 34: Outcome of severe damage to the central nervous system* (pp. 191–213). Amsterdam: Elsevier-Excerpta Medica-North-Holland.

Shalet, S. M., Beardwell, C. G., Tworney, J. H., Jones, P. H. M., & Pearson, D. (1977). Endocrine function following the treatment of acute leukemia in childhood. *Journal of Pediatrics, 90*, 920–923.

Shere, M. O. (1957). The socio-emotional development of the twin who has cerebral palsy. *Cerebral Palsy Review, 18,* 16–18.

Shontz, F. C. (1971). Physical disability and personality. In W. S. Neff (Ed.), *Rehabilitation psychology* (pp. 33–37). Washington, DC: American Psychological Association.

Shore, M. F., & Goldston, S. E. (1978). Mental health aspects of pediatric care. Historical review and current status. In P. R. Magreb (Ed.), *Psychological management of pediatric problems: Vol. 1. Early life conditions and chronic diseases* (pp. 15–31). Baltimore: University Park Press.

Siegel, F. S., Barlow, B., Fisch, R. O., & Anderson, V. E. (1968). School behavior profile ratings of phenylketonuric children. *American Journal of Mental Deficiency, 72,* 937–943.

Siegel, L. J. (1974). Preparation of children for hospitalization: A selected review of the literature. *Journal of Pediatric Psychology, 56,* 26–30.

Silverberg, E. (1982). Cancer Statistics, 1982. *Ca-A Cancer Journal for Clinicians, 32,* (1), 15–31.

Simeonsson, R., Buckley, L., & Monson, L. (1979). Conceptions of illness causality in hospitalized children. *Journal of Pediatric Psychology, 4,* 77–84.

Simpson, H. (1980). Asthma in childhood. In D. C. Flenley (Ed.), *Recent advances in respiratory medicine* (pp. 153–167). Edinburgh & London: Churchill-Livingstone.

Sipowicz, R. R., & Vernon, D. T. A. (1965). Psychological responses of children to hospitalization. *American Journal of Diseases of Children, 109,* 228–231.

Skipper, J. K., & Leonard, R. C. (1968). Children, stress and hospitalization: A field experiment. *Journal of Health and Social Behavior, 9,* 275–281.

Slavin, L. A., O'Malley, J. E., Koocher, G., & Foster, D. J. (1982). Communication of the cancer diagnosis to pediatric patients: Impact on long-term adjustment. *American Journal of Psychiatry, 139*(2), 179–183.

Smith, I., Lobascher, M. E., Stevenson, J. E., Wolff, O. H., Schmidt, H., Grübel-Kaiser, S., & Bickel, H. (1978). Effects of stopping low-phenylalanine diet on intellectual progress of children with phenylketonuria. *British Medical Journal, 2,* 723–726.

Smith, I., Lobascher, M., & Wolff, O. H. (1973). Factors influencing outcome in early treatment of phenylketonuria. In J. W. T. Seakins, R. A. Saunder, & C. Toothill (Eds.), *Treatment of inborn errors of metabolism* (pp. 41–49). Edinburgh & London: Churchill-Livingstone.

Smith, I., & Wolff, O. H. (1974). Natural history of phenylketonuria and influences of early treatment. *Lancet, 2,* 540–544.

Smith, R. (1981). Health education by children for children. *British Medical Journal, 283,* 782–783.

Soni, S. S., Marten, G. W., Pitner, S. E., Duenas, D. A., & Powazek, M. (1975). Effects of central nervous system irradiation on neuropsychologic functioning of children with acute lymphocytic leukemia. *New England Journal of Medicine, 293,* 113–118.

Spinetta, J. J., & Maloney, L. J. (1975). Death anxiety in the outpatient leukemic child. *Pediatrics, 56,* 1034–1037.

Spinetta, J. J., & Maloney, L. T. (1978). The child with cancer: Patterns of communication and denial. *Journal of Consulting and Clinical Psychology, 46,* 1540–1541.

Spinetta, J. J., Rigler, D., & Karon, M. (1973). Anxiety in the dying child. *Pediatrics, 52,* 841–845.

Spinetta, J. J., Rigler, D., & Karon, M. (1974). Personal space as a measure of a dying child's sense of isolation. *Journal of Consulting and Clinical Psychology, 42,* 751–757.

Spinetta, P. D., & Spinetta, J. J. (1980). Teacher's appraisal: The child with cancer in school. *American Journal of Pediatric Hematology/Oncology, 2,* 89–94.

Stacey, M., Dearden, R., Pill, R., & Robinson, D. (1970). *Hospitals, children and their families: The report of a pilot study.* London: Routledge and Kegan Paul.

Starr, P. (1978). Self-esteem and behavioral functioning of teenagers with oral-facial clefts. *Rehabilitation Literature, 39,* 233–235.

Starte, G. D. (1978). Influence of illness on developmental progress in children under 2. *Journal of the Royal College of General Practice, 28,* 273–277.

Stehbens, J. A. (1983). A statistical quirk? Reply to Kellerman, Moss and Siegel. *Journal of Pediatric Psychology, 8*(4), 379–382.

Stehbens, J. A., Ford, M. E., Kisker, C. T., Clarke, W. R., & Strayer, F. (1981). WISC-R verbal performance discrepancies in pediatric cancer patients. *Journal of Pediatric Psychology, 6,* 61–68.

Stehbens, J. A., Kisker, C. T., & Wilson, B. K. (1983). Achievement and intelligence test-retest performance in pediatric cancer patients at diagnosis and one year later. *Journal of Pediatric Psychology, 8*(1), 47–56.

Stein, R. E. K., & Jessop, D. J. (1984). Relationship between health status and psychological adjustment among children with chronic conditions. *Pediatrics, 73,* 169–174.

Stein, S. P., & Charles, E. (1971). Emotional factors in juvenile diabetes mellitus: A study of early life expectancies of adolescent diabetics. *American Journal of Psychiatry, 128,* 700–704.

Steinhauer, P. D., Mushin, D. N., & Rae-Grant, Q. (1974). Psychological aspects of chronic illness. *Pediatric Clinics of North America, 21,* 825–840.

Steinhausen, H. C. (1975). A psychoclinical investigation in adult hemophiliacs. *Journal of Psychosomatic Research, 19,* 295–302.

Steinhauser, H., Borner, S., & Koepp, P. (1977). The personality of juvenile diabetes. In Z. Laron (Ed.), *Pediatric and adolescent endocrinology: Vol. 3.* Basel: Karger.

Stevenson, J. E., Hawcroft, J., Lobascher, M., Smith, I., Wolff, O. H., & Graham, P. J. (1979). Behavioural deviance in children with early treated PKU. *Archives of Disease in Childhood, 54,* 14–18.

Steward, M. S., & Regalbuto, G. (1975). Do doctors know what children know? *American Journal of Orthopsychiatry, 45,* 146–149.

Steward, M. S., & Steward, D. S. (1981). Children's conceptions of medical procedures. In R. Bibace & M. E. Walsh (Eds.), *Children's conceptions of health, illness and bodily functions* (pp. 67–84). San Francisco: Jossey-Bass.

Stewart, W. (1967). The unmet needs of children. *Pediatrics, 39,* 157–160.

Stewart-Brown, S., Haslum, M., & Butler, N. (1983). Evidence for increasing prevalence of diabetes mellitus in childhood. *British Medical Journal, 286,* 1855–1857.

Stott, A. (1966). *The social adjustment of children* (3rd ed). London: University of London Press.

Straus, M. A., & Tallman, I. (1971). SIMFAM: A technique for observational measurement and experimental study of families. In J. Aldous, (Ed.), *Family problem solving* (pp. 379–438). Hillsdale, IL: Dryden Press.

Strickland, B. R. (1978). Internal–external expectancies and health-related behaviors. *Journal of Consulting and Clinical Psychology, 46,* 1192–1211.

Strowig, S. (1982). Patient education: A model for autonomous decision-making and deliberate action in diabetes self-management. *Medical Clinics of North America, 66,* 6, 1293–1307.

Stubblefield, R. (1974). Psychiatric complications of chronic illness in children. In J. A. Downey & N. L. Low (Eds.), *The child with disabling illness.* Philadelphia: W. B. Saunders.

Sullivan, B. J. (1979). Adjustment in diabetic adolescent girls: I. Development of the diabetic adjustment Scale; II, Adjustment, self-esteem, and depression in diabetic adolescent girls. *Psychosomatic Medicine, 41,* 119–138.

Susman, E. J., Hollenbeck, A. R., Nannis, E. D., & Strope, B. E. (1980). A developmental perspective on psychosocial aspects of childhood cancer. In J. L. Schulman & M. J. Kupst (Eds.), *The child with cancer: Clinical approaches to psychosocial care—Research in psychosocial aspects* (pp. 129–142). Springfield, IL: C. C. Thomas.

Sussman, M. B. (1966). Sociological theory and deafness: Problems and prospects. *ASHA: Journal of American Speech and Hearing Association, 8,* 303–307.

Sutherland, I., Hudson, F. P., & Hawcroft, J. (1978). MRC/DHSS *Phenylketonuria Register Newsletter* No. 5.

Swift, C. R., Seidman, F., & Stein, H. (1967). Adjustment problems in juvenile diabetes. *Psychosomatic Medicine, 29,* 555–571.

Tait, C. D., & Ascher, R. C. (1955). Inside-of-the-body test. *Psychosomatic Medicine, 17,* 139–148.

Tamaroff, M., Miller, D. R., Murphy, M. L., Salwen, R., Ghavimi, M. D., & Nir, Y. (1982). Immediate and long-term post-therapy neuropsychologic performance in children with acute lymphoblastic leukemia treated without central nervous radiation. *Journal of Pediatrics, 101,* 524–529.

Tattersall, R. B., & Jackson, J. G. L. (1982). Social and emotional complications of diabetes. In H. Keen & J. Jarrett (Eds.), *Complications of diabetes* (pp. 271–285). London: Edward Arnold.

Tavormina, J. B., Kastner, L. S., Slater, P. M., & Watt, S. L. (1976). Chronically sick children: A psychological and emotionally deviant population. *Journal of Abnormal Child Psychology, 4,* 99–110.

Taylor, D. C., & Falconer, M. A. (1968). Clinical socio-economic and psychological change after temporal lobectomy for epilepsy. *British Journal of Psychiatry, 114,* 1247–1261.

Teagarden, F. M. (1939). The intelligence of diabetic children with some case reports. *Journal of Applied Psychology, 23,* 337–351.

Tew, B. J., Payne, J., & Laurence, K. M. (1974). Must a family with a handicapped child be a handicapped family? *Developmental Medicine and Child Neurology, 16* (Suppl. 32), 95–98.

Thompson, C. W., Garner, A. M., & Partridge, J. W. (1969). Sick? or diabetic? A research report. *Diabetes Bulletin, 45,* 2–3.

Thornes, R. (1983). Parental access and family facilities in children's wards in England. *British Medical Journal, 287,* 190–192.

Tiller, J. W. G., Ekert, H., & Rickards, W. S. (1977). Family reactions in childhood acute lymphoblastic leukaemia in remission. *Australian Paediatric Journal, 13*, 176–181.

Travis, G. (1976). *Chronic illness in childhood: Its impact on child and family*. Stanford, CA: Stanford University Press.

Tropauer, A., Franz, M. N., & Dilgard, V. W. (1970). Psychological aspects of the care of children with cystic fibrosis. *American Journal of Diseases of Children, 119*, 424–432.

Turk, J. (1964). Impact of cystic fibrosis on family functioning. *Pediatrics, 34*, 67–71.

Twaddle, V., Britton, P. G., Craft, A. C., Noble, T. C., & Kernahan, J. (1983). Intellectual function after treatment for leukaemia or solid tumours. *Archives of Disease in Childhood, 58*, 949–952.

Vandeman, P. (1963). Termination of dietary treatment for phenylketonuria. *American Journal of Diseases of Children, 106*, 492–495.

Varonier, H. S. (1970). Prevalence of allergy among children and adolescents in Geneva, Switzerland. *Respiration, 27*, 115–120.

Vaughan, G. (1957). Children in hospital. *Lancet, 272*, 1117–1120.

Vernick, J., & Karon, J. (1965). Who's afraid of death on a leukemia ward? *American Journal of Diseases of Children, 109*, 393–397.

Vernon, D. T. A. (1973). Use of modeling to modify children's responses to a natural potentially stressful situation. *Journal of Applied Psychology, 58*, 351–357.

Vernon, D. T. A,. & Bailey, W. (1974). The use of motion pictures in the psychological preparation of children for induction of anesthesia. *Anesthesiology, 40*, 68–72.

Vernon, D. T., Foley, J. M., & Schulman, J. L. (1967). Effect of mother–child separation and birth order on young children's responses to two potentially stressful situations. *Journal of Personality and Social Psychology, 5*, 162–174.

Vernon, D., & Schulman, J. (1964). Hospitalization as a source of psychological benefit to children. *Pediatrics, 34*, 694–696.

Vernon, D., Schulman, J., & Foley, J. (1966). Changes in children's behavior after hospitalization. *American Journal of Diseases of Children, 111*, 581–593.

Vernon, M. (1969). *Multiple handicapped deaf children: Medical education and psychological considerations. Council for Exceptional Children, research monograph*. Washington, DC: Council for Exceptional Children.

Verzosa, M. S., Aur, R. J. A., Simon, J. V., Hustu, H. O., & Pinkel, D. P. (1976). Five years after central nervous system irradiation of children with leukemia. *International Journal of Radiation Oncology, Biology, Physics, 1*, 209–215.

Vignos, P. Jr., Thompson, H. M., Katz, W., Moskowitz, F. W., Fink, W., & Svec, K. H. (1972). Comprehensive care and psychological factors in rehabilitation in chronic rheumatoid arthritis: A controlled study. *Journal of Chronic Diseases, 22*, 457–467.

Waechter, E. H. (1971). Children's awareness of fatal illness. *American Journal of Nursing*, 1168–1172.

Waisbren, S. E., Schnell, R. R., & Levy, H. L. (1980). Diet termination in children with phenylketonuria: A review of psychological assessments used to determine outcome. *Journal of Inherited Metabolic Disease*, 149–153.

Wallach, M. A., & Kogan, N. (1965). *Modes of thinking in young children*. New York: Holt, Rinehart & Winston.

Wallston, B. S., & Wallston, K. A. (1978). Locus of control and health: A review of the literature. *Health Education Monographs, 6*, 107–117.

Wallston, B. S., Wallston, K. A., Kaplan, G. D., & Maides, S. A. (1976). Development and validation of the Health Locus of Control (HLC) scale. *Journal of Consulting and Clinical Psychology, 44*, 580–585.

Wallston, K. A., & Wallston, B. S. (1981). Who is responsible for your health? The construct of health locus of control. In G. Sanders & J. Suls (Eds.), *Social psychology of health and illness* (pp. 65–95). Hillsdale, NJ: Lawrence Erlbaum.

Ward, F. W., & Bower, B. D. (1978). A study of certain social aspects of epilepsy in childhood. *Developmental Medicine and Child Neurology, 20*(1), 1–63.

Wechsler, D. (1974). *Manual for the Wechsler Intelligence Scale for Children—Revised.* New York: Psychological Corporation.

Wedell-Monnig, J., & Lumley, J. M. (1980). Child deafness and mother–child interaction. *Child Development, 51*, 766–774.

Weinberg, N., & Santana, R. (1978). Comic books: Champions of the disabled stereotype. *Rehabilitation Literature, 39*(11–12), 327–331.

Weir, K., & Duveen, G. (1981). Further development and validation of the prosocial behavior questionnaire for use by teachers. *Journal of Child Psychology and Psychiatry and Allied Disciplines, 22*, 41, 357–374.

Weiss, E. (1950). Psychosomatic aspects of certain allergic disorders. *International Archives of Allergy, 1*, 4–28.

Werner, H. (1948). *Comparative psychology of mental development.* New York: Science Editions.

Whitt, J. K., Dykstra, W., & Taylor, C. A. (1979). Children's conceptions of illness and cognitive development: Implications for pediatric practitioners. *Clinical Pediatrics, 18*, 327–339.

Williams, C. (1970). Some psychiatric observations on a group of maladjusted deaf children. *Journal of Child Psychology and Psychiatry and Allied Disciplines, 11*, 1–18.

Williams, H. E., & McNicol, K. N. (1969). Prevalence, natural history and relationship of wheezy bronchitis and asthma in children. An epidemiological survey. *British Medical Journal, 4*, 321–325.

Williams, H. E., & McNicol, K. N. (1975). The spectrum of asthma in children. *Pediatric Clinics of North America, 22*, 43–52.

Williamson, M., Koch, R., & Berlow, S. (1979). Diet discontinuation in phenylketonuria. *Pediatrics, 63*, 823–824.

Willoughby, M. L. N. (1973). Disorders of the blood and reticulo-endothelial system. In J. O. Forfar & G. C. Arneil (Eds.), *Textbook of paediatrics* (pp. 935–982). London: Churchill-Livingstone. 3rd edition.

Wing, J. K., Cooper, J. E., & Sartorius, N. (1974). *Measurement and classification of psychiatry symptoms.* Cambridge, England: Cambridge University Press.

Wisely, D. W., Masur, F. T., & Morgan, S. B. (1983). Psychological aspects of severe burn injuries in children. *Health Psychology, 2*, 45–72.

Wold, D. A., & Townes, B. D. (1969). The adjustment of siblings to childhood leukaemia. *Childhood Coordinator, 18*, 155–160.

Wolfer, J. A., & Visintainer, M. A. (1979). Prehospital psychological preparation for tonsillectomy patients: Effects on children's and parent's adjustment. *Pediatrics, 64*(5), 646–655.

Wood, A. C., Friedman, C. J., & Steisel, I. M. (1967). Psychosocial factors in phenylketonuria. *American Journal of Orthopsychiatry, 37*, 671–679.

Woolf, L. I., Griffiths, R., Moncreiff, A., Coates, S., & Dillistone, F. (1958). The dietary treatment of phenylketonuria. *Archives of Disease in Childhood, 33*, 31–45.

Wright, B. (1960). *Physical disability: A psychological approach.* New York: Harper & Row.

Wright, L. (1975). Pediatric psychology and problems of physical health. *Journal of Clinical and Child Psychology*, (Fall), 13–15.

Zartler, A. S., & Sassaman, E. (1981). Linguistic development in PKU. *Journal of Pediatrics, 99*(3), 501.

Author Index

Cassel, J.C., 126–128, 166
Cassell, S., 46, 167
Cayler, G.C., 66, 167
Cenlec, P., 119, 167
Centrewall, C., 85, 167
Centrewall, W.R., 85, 167
Cernek, D., 119, 167
Chadwick, O., 64, 65, 71, 188
Chandler, B.C., 9, 62, 101, 166
Chandler, M.J., 4, 7, 187
Chang, P., 92, 93, 167, 171
Charles, E., 98, 190
Chase, G.A., 87, 178
Cherry, T., 106, 107, 110, 184
Chess, S., 171
Chessells, J., 130, 132, 144, 168
Childs, B., 87, 178
Ching, A.Y.T., 123, 169, 181
Chodoff, P., 147, 168, 172
Christ, A.E., 188
Claiborne, R., 175
Clare, A.W., 147, 168
Clarke, W.R., 140, 142, 190
Cloup, I., 117, 179
Coates, S., 85, 194
Cobb, B., 79, 168
Coburn, C., 103, 170
Coddington, R.D., 98, 124–126, 168
Cohen, D., 83, 179
Cohen, L.D., 123, 178
Cohen, S.E., 66, 164, 165
Cohen, S.I., 118, 168
Cole, P., 131, 163
Colle, E., 96, 184
Collier, A.M., 126–128, 166
Collier, B.N., 103, 168
Collins, J.L., 66, 168
Comaroff, J., 25, 133, 147, 168, 180
Conley, J.A., 92, 171
Conners, C.K., 71, 168
Cook, S.D., 25, 35, 168
Coolidge, J.C., 123, 168
Cooper, J.E., 147, 193
Cooper, J.S., 121, 122, 129, 164
Cooper, P.F., 67, 174
Copeland, D.R., 135, 136, 151, 178
Coutts, J.M.J., 92, 177
Cowen, E.L., 62, 65, 154, 168
Craft, A.C., 140, 143, 145, 192

Craig, O., 63, 168
Crain, A.R., 111, 168
Crider, C., 22, 157, 168
Crisco, J.J., 134—136, 150, 183
Crouthamel, C., 68, 173
Crowe, E.A., 66, 165
Cumming, G., 116, 182
Cutter, F., 123, 168

Davidson, A.N., 169
Davidson, F.R., 151, 167
Davidson, W., 83, 87, 174
Davie, R., 41, 159, 168
Davis, D.M., 94, 110, 168
Davis, F., 14, 168
Davis, J.A., 169
Davis, J.H., 183
Dawson, B., 121, 182
Dearden, R., 43, 190
Dekker, B., 118, 169
Delbridge, L., 99, 110, 169
Demb, N., 78
Denning, C., 14, 184
Department of Health and Social Se-
    curity, 169
de Vries, K., 118, 169
Dichiro, G., 138, 183
Dikmen, S., 64, 169
Dilgard, V.W., 63, 67, 192
Dillistone, F., 85, 194
Dimock, H.G., 48, 169
di Sant'Agnese, P., 23, 166
Divitto, B., 66, 169, 173
Dobbing, J., 65, 138, 169
Dobson, J.C., 85, 87, 169, 177
Doershuk, C.F., 68, 178
Doise, W., 156, 183
Dolger, H., 110, 171
Donker, D.M., 93, 169
Dornbusch, S.M., 99, 186
Douglas, J.W.B., 7, 8, 43–45, 50, 61,
    169, 185
Downey, J.A., 191
Downing, R.W., 71, 169
Drash, A., 103, 170
Dreher, M., 112, 188
Drotar, D., 68, 178
Dubo, S., 32, 123, 169

Subject Index